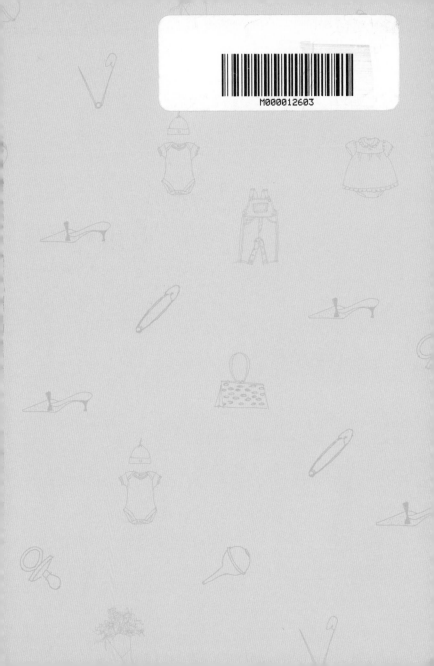

Milk It

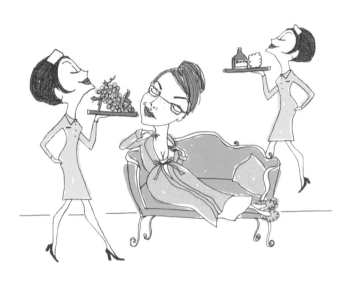

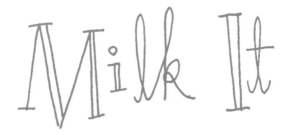

Milk It

How to Get More than a Baby out of the Next Nine Months

Kate Hodson

Illustrations *by* Alanna Cavanagh

CHRONICLE BOOKS
SAN FRANCISCO

Library of Congress Cataloging-in-Publication Data available.

ISBN-10: 0-8118-5311-X
ISBN-13: 978-0-8118-5311-8

Manufactured in China.

Designed by Jacob T. Gardner

Distributed in Canada by Raincoast Books
9050 Shaughnessy Street
Vancouver, British Columbia V6P 6E5

10 9 8 7 6 5 4 3 2 1

Chronicle Books LLC
85 Second Street
San Francisco, California 94105

www.chroniclebooks.com

To Phoebe and Molly

TABLE *of* *CONTENTS*

INTRODUCTION

I love being pregnant. You can eat what you like. People are really nice to you. And then, at the end of it all, you get a big, fat baby to play with. It's a lot of fun.

Most of the time.

Unfortunately, pregnancy does have its smattering of oddities and inconveniences. There are some dodgy physical symptoms that pop up now and again. Then there's the money you have to spend on a whole new super-stretchy wardrobe. And, of course, it's really hard to party like it's 1999 when you have a belly as firm and as round as a freakishly large gourd. Perhaps your pregnancy isn't exactly turning out to be the free-wheeling, all-you-can-eat lark you were hoping for. If that's the case, you have only one course of action. You owe it to yourself to seek out every last perk of bellydom, and take advantage of all that your newly pregnant life has to offer.

So alongside the books that tell you how your fetus is growing (like a creature possessed, apparently) and what to eat (lots), here's one that will help you make the most of what used to be called a *confinement*, but now may be more accurately termed a well-deserved opportunity for *self-edification* and *personal fulfillment*.

Having a baby is not just about replicating your more attractive physical characteristics, or about taking a really long time off work. You are doing a Very Important Thing. The child you are carrying could be destined for greatness. There are all kinds of diseases left to cure, and why shouldn't socialism be a viable political alternative? Thanks to you and your exceptional pregnancy skills, world peace could be a real possibility in the not-too-distant future. At the very least, you're keeping the designers at Baby Gap gainfully employed *and* giving your mother something other than your career (stagnant) and your partner (unkempt) to focus on. So while your new task is ostensibly to nurture that embryo or fetus (or whatever developmental stage your baby-to-be is at), there's no harm in diversifying a little and working the system to your own personal benefit.

And a system there surely is. There is nothing easy and carefree about being pregnant. Oh, no. For one thing, people expect an awful lot of pregnant women. There's no smoking or drinking, and lewd behavior in public is definitely frowned upon. You have to eat right, look presentable, and be serene and glowing at all times. You are expected to take exemplary care of yourself for the health of your future child. And you have to do it all under public scrutiny. It's quite the responsibility. Which makes it all the more important that you seek out the bonuses that come with pregnancy, and milk them for all they're worth.

Rest assured, it's all good, harmless fun. Know that you can be bad tempered, lazy, and demanding and still have a cheerful and contented baby. You can indulge yourself in millions of small ways and still have a cute kid. So you make yourself look a little bit more pregnant just to get a little bit more sympathy. So what? It doesn't mean that you're destined to be a bad mother. Just a very smart one.

Apart from anything else, this is *the very last time in your life* when it's all about you. As soon as that baby emerges from your crotch and hauls his way up to your burgeoning boobs, lips a-smacking, a glint in his eye, you'll know that your self-indulgent, selfish, and self-centered life is well and truly over.

So enjoy your pregnancy. Allow yourself the pleasure of being big, bad, bold, and bossy. Change doctors on a whim, force old people out of their seats on the bus, snap at strangers who touch your tummy, and take permanent control of the TV remote. Make up for all the things pregnancy forbids, prevents, or otherwise renders not much fun by devising for yourself some new recreational activities that make you smile, lift your spirits, and make you thoroughly glad to be pregnant. So it's a little underhanded. Again, so what? That's what the perks of pregnancy are all about.

A CAVEAT OF SORTS

For the sake of argument, I've assumed that you, the pregnant reader of this book are female, and that (A) you have a partner, and (B) your partner, the other parent of your child, is male. Clearly, this is a generalization, and generalizations by definition do not hold true for everybody. Families come in all shapes, sizes, and sexes. My assumption is simply a writer's convenience and is not intended as any kind of political or moral statement. Far from it. In fact, my sense is that if your partner is another woman, you probably won't have to work quite so hard to get the extra pampering that you deserve (other women being typically more empathetic toward the pregnantly challenged).

I've also made the assumption that you'll be having your baby in some kind of hospital setting—another example of wanton generalization—mainly because this is what most people do. Many other options are available to you, of course, and I encourage you to seek out birth centers, midwives, or bathtubs, and have the kind of birth experience you've always wanted. It seems that there are as many ways to give birth (or at least variations on a basic theme) as there are to get pregnant (likewise), and only you know what's going to work best for you.

I had both of my babies in a hospital setting and ended up having an epidural on both occasions. When I had my first baby, I was naïve and exhausted and, as it transpired, I had larked off in my childbirth class one time too many. Once at the hospital (to be induced just four days after my due date, for reasons that still confound me), I simply got swept along by the tide of medical intervention. When I gave birth to my second, even larger, child, it appeared that, coincidentally, I had again failed to pay attention in my childbirth refresher class (particularly the bit about using slow and regular breathing to lessen the mounting sense of panic engendered by the rapid onset of labor and what turned out to be dilation from three to ten centimeters in about forty-five minutes). Just for the record, it is entirely possible to get an epidural when you're ten centimeters dilated, if you yell long and loud enough.

At this point, seeing as we're already talking about doctors and hospitals and fantastic anesthesiologists, I'd also like to acknowledge the members of the medical profession, mainly because I'm related to a couple of them, and I know firsthand that they are genuinely kind and caring people and not the unsympathetic, self-absorbed slackers that certain chapters of this book might suggest. I received excellent care during my pregnancies and the birth of (especially) my second child, and I'd definitely mention the name of the obstetrical practice I visited throughout my pregnancy, the hospital where she was born, and the doctor who delivered her, if only I could be sure that they'd welcome an endorsement from such a dubious source.

Finally, I've assumed that your baby will be entering the world via the usual channel (i.e., the vagina), again because this is how the majority of them get here, and (not to get embarrassingly personal or anything) because it is representative of my own experience. But, of course, babies can be born in all kinds of ways, and (to my limited medical knowledge) through at least two different exit routes. Listen to your instincts (and maybe even your childbirth class instructor), and you'll inevitably do what is right for you and your baby.

Deciding to have a baby

How to get your partner on board, as it were

Since time began, there have been women who have thought it a terribly clever idea to get themselves pregnant without the prior knowledge and consent of their husband/boyfriend/casual pickup. In fact, this idea is not terribly clever at all and only works if all you want is a baby. If you're looking for stability in your relationship, or at least

a second date, you should remember that men are like women in many respects (notable exceptions include the pride with which they pass gas in public and their limitless appreciation of toilet humor) and don't respond well to being duped. If nothing else, it is recommended that you tell the daddy-to-be that he might soon be a daddy;

or that you have Big Plans for his sperm; or that you have decided that, instead of grouting the bathroom this weekend, the two of you will be making a baby.

The best-case scenario for a harmonious and long-lasting relationship is, of course, to arrive jointly at the decision to procreate. Which is all fine and dandy, except that it assumes both parties have already acknowledged that the concept of parenthood is a subject up for debate. And herein lies the problem.

While you and your partner may be of one mind when it comes to ordering Thai instead of Chinese takeout or vacationing in Hawaii as opposed to Florida, it's unlikely that the strange yet delightful idea to have a baby will strike you both simultaneously and with equal force. On the contrary, it seems that in most relationships there is one person who has the baby idea first (let's call this person the *woman*) and one person who is instantly suspicious of her suggestion (hereafter referred to as the *man*). In order to further the species, the woman must overcome the often-slender objections ("I'm way too young/old/scared to have kids") offered up by the man, usually by pretending to listen with deep understanding while thinking of something else entirely.

Although the woman's desire to procreate usually prevails, this process may be expedited by following the three steps outlined below:

STEP 1:
INTRODUCE THE IDEA.
(Either A. by example)

Congratulations. You may consider yourself halfway pregnant if you and your partner have a couple of close friends, preferably in a relationship, preferably with each other, who are themselves expecting a baby. It is now only a matter of time before you get the green light on your own pregnancy. The speed with which this happens is directly proportional to how comfortable this other couple is with the journey to parenthood.

Ideally, the mother-to-be (a.k.a. your new best friend) should be a glowing example of pregnant perfection who wears super-cute maternity clothes showcasing a neat and tidy bump (the exact size and shape of a bowling ball, or basketball, or whatever kind of ball your partner fixates on most). The father-to-be should be a healthily masculine, beer-swilling, ESPN-watching kind of chap who finds strange fascination in all things fetal, including childbirth classes and maternity bras, while still enjoying his Monday Night Football and Friday Night Out with the Boys.

Know that this unlikely and, let's face it, highly annoying couple holds your fast pass to Labor and Delivery (by way of Expensive Last-Minute Weekend Getaway and Way Too Much Wine at Dinner), so plan on spending a lot of time with them, even if their unnatural perfection (and any ensuing smugness) pushes you to the brink of prepregnancy nausea. Because at some wondrous point—ideally before they ask you to film the birth of their baby—it will occur to your partner that this whole pregnancy thing isn't such a bad idea, and wouldn't it be kind of neat to have one of those baby-type things in our house too? Best of all, he will think that this is entirely His Own Idea, which is, of course, the optimal situation.

NOTE: It's vital that you adopt these people as your role models before they actually have their child. Wait too long and the whole exhausting truth about new babies will become horribly apparent.

If you don't have a pair of pregnant friends to hold up as shining examples of well-adjusted parents-to-be, you have no choice but to be completely truthful with your partner. Obviously, under normal circumstances, this would be the last resort. These are *exceptional* circumstances, however, and while subtlety (of the underhanded and strategic variety) may be your preferred approach to getting your own way in most situations, there is nothing understated about babies. They yell, their stuff takes up a lot of room, and they poop their pants in public. It's almost impossible to sneak something like that into an everyday conversation.

Your best shot at success is to be straightforward (which will earn you points), but in an ego-stroking kind of way (resulting in even more points). Instead of simply saying, "I want to have a baby," consider saying something more along the lines of "I'd like to have your baby," or "I can't think of anybody who would make a better dad," or "When I look at you I see the future," depending on your threshold for saccharine. Then at least your partner will feel somewhat integral to the whole glorious undertaking.

STEP 2:

PRESENT SUPPORTING ARGUMENTS.

However you introduce the idea of procreation, you will most likely be required (by elderly relatives if not by your somewhat baffled partner) to provide evidence showing why now is the perfect time to throw away those contraceptive pills and embrace pregnancy, parenthood, and other things beginning with p.

The following are commonly understood to be perfectly acceptable, if not downright vital, reasons to make a baby. Feel free to use them to further your cause:

1. **YOUR STRONG RELATIONSHIP (RECENTLY CONFIRMED BY YOUR $19.95 ONLINE ASTROLOGICAL COUPLE'S PROFILE)**

2. **YOUR FINANCIAL STABILITY (YOUR 1986 JETTA IS ALMOST PAID FOR.)**

3. **THE EXTRA ROOM/CLOSET/DRAWER SPACE IN YOUR APARTMENT (AS LONG AS YOU CAN CURB YOUR HANDBAG AND FLIP-FLOP OBSESSIONS)**

4. **YOUR HITHERTO UNTAPPED TALENT FOR KNITTING SMALL GARMENTS (WELL, HOW DIFFICULT CAN IT REALLY BE?)**

5. **THE FACT THAT HIS STRONG TEETH AND GOOD HAIR WILL OFFSET YOUR FAMILY HISTORY OF KLEPTOMANIA AND THE LARGISH BOTTOMS ON YOUR MOTHER'S SIDE (JUST KEEPING THE GENE POOL NICE AND CLEAN)**

STEP 3:

CLOSE THE DEAL.

This is usually a no-brainer, since few men will turn down the prospect of more sex.

Trying to get pregnant

As soon as a potential pregnancy is on the table, or hopefully somewhere else a little easier on your back, your partner will start to cycle through a series of emotions. This sequence typically commences with Ashen-Faced Horror, moves fairly rapidly through Night Sweats, Morning Sickness, and Terminal Resignation, before settling on Testicular Pride.

At the same time, you will be seized by an incredible desire to tell everyone you know that you are officially "fertile ground," or something similarly euphemistic. And why shouldn't you? After all, this is big news. Since you can't yet tell people that you are actually "expecting a happy event" (or something similarly euphemistic), this is the most exciting thing you have going on at the moment—especially if it's the end of February or early November or one of those boring nonvacation times of the year. But on behalf of your friends as well as your wiser self, I urge you not to follow this verbal path. There are some really good reasons why.

REALLY GOOD REASON #1:
IT'S TOO MUCH INFORMATION.

Picture the scene. You and a coworker are enjoying a couple of low-fat chai lattes at your favorite beverage emporium. You've dished about your relationship, you've gossiped about her mother-in-law, and now it's your turn again to be indiscreet.

YOU SAY: Matt and I are trying to get pregnant.

YOU SEE: Soft fuzzy hair, big blue eyes, hours spent shopping for baby clothes.

YOUR FRIEND HEARS: Matt and I are trying to get pregnant.

YOUR FRIEND SEES: Matt and you having sex.

However you try to pitch the concept of procreation, there's no doubt in anybody's mind about what the process entails. This visual imagery may be fine for very close friends or your unusually open-minded parents, but please consider the digestive tracts of your more sensitive acquaintances.

REALLY GOOD REASON #2:
IT'S TOO SOON.

You may turn out to be the single most fertile woman in the world, falling pregnant while fully clothed after one smoldering glance from your partner. But if your potential to conceive is less than immaculate (and it probably is, considering that even a woman in her early twenties has only a 50 percent chance of conceiving in any one cycle), there may be months and months between (**A**) deciding to have a baby and (**B**) a positive pregnancy test. If you are currently at point (**A**), even your gynecologist doesn't need a blow-by-blow account of your activities in order to hasten your arrival at (**B**). A simple mention that you're trying to conceive, casually thrown out at your next visit, will suffice. And although you may be tempted, making a special appointment at this point in order to subject your doctor to a bunch of pregnancy- and childbirth-related questions is simply unnecessary and, worse, may even prejudice him or her against you. And never forget who has the power to order the epidural you always said you didn't want.

REALLY GOOD REASON #3:
YOU'LL GET TOO MANY QUESTIONS.

The more people you tell, the more people you'll have watching your waistline, monitoring your eating habits, and counting the number of trips per hour you make to the bathroom. And then there are those people who think of themselves as refreshingly forthright when really they're just rude and unpleasant—those people who feel obliged to come right out with "Are you pregnant yet?" or "How's the whole conception thing going?" to which you should probably say something noncommittal and conversation stopping like "We'll probably start a family in a year or two" or "Matt hates kids."

Breaking the news to your partner

How to drop the bombshell for minimal devastation

Let's assume for a minute that you and your chosen life partner have made a joint and mutually acceptable decision to increase the world's population by one smallish infant. Together, you have considered important things like the size of your abode, the size of your income, and your tolerance for diapering, and you are agreed. You are now officially trying for a baby.

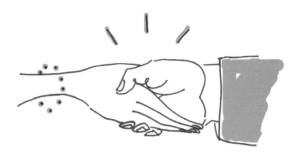

You, the childbearing half in this scheme, start taking prenatal vitamins and throw away (in a gesture as dramatic as it is symbolic) your contraceptive pills. Your partner, in an effort to compensate for his (let's face it) much smaller role, struts around feeling both powerful and somehow taken advantage of, all at the same time.

Then the pair of you proceed to do what you need to do, at appropriate intervals, and with the necessary frequency. At some point you figure that things might have worked, that you might have become a vessel, or up the duff, or however you care to put it. You rush out and purchase a pregnancy test (at great and seemingly unwarranted expense, until the result is positive, when it suddenly seems like such a small price to pay). Then you pee on a stick.

It appears that the most amazing thing has happened. You're thrilled and delighted, nervous and excited, horrified and appalled. It's time to share the news with the now second most important person in your life. Why, then, do you feel like you're confessing to having done A Very Bad Thing, like going over the limit on your credit card again, or sending an unsolicited flirtatious e-mail to an old boyfriend? Because, even though you decided together that you wanted to start a family, even though he knew that nobody in this little tryst was practicing safe sex, even though he's been sleeping with a woman of childbearing age, you know he's going to be more than a little surprised. Ultimately, of course, he'll be delighted. He'll take personal pride in the speed and accuracy of his sperm. He'll enjoy the glory that's reflected in your growing belly. But right now, it's the thing that he thought would never happen.

He's got a girl pregnant.

Without doubt, this is news that needs to be relayed very gently and very calmly, and in a very specific manner. For maximum success (i.e., minimum irreversible emotional fallout), consider taking the following steps:

ASSUME POSITIONS.

HIM: Seated.

YOU: At least an arm's length away (in the event of a dangerous reflexive lunge).

STEP 2:
PREPARE OPENING GAMBIT.

Choose your words very carefully. It's critical that you get your phrasing right, from the second you open your mouth to the moment you pick him up off the floor. In fact, from this point on, everything you say (or don't say) and do (or don't) should inform him, explicitly or subliminally, that you are in control of the situation, and that even though you are pregnant, *you will still be taking care of him.* Men respond well to this, the big dweebs. Try one of these conversational openers:

WHAT YOU SAY: "Honey, we've got big news."
HOW YOU SAY IT: Encouraging. Maternal.
RATIONALE: This is a good one. It's warm and friendly, the "we've" hints at something you've achieved together (a clue to the clueless), and nobody can deny that what you're about to say is *big*.

WHAT YOU SAY: "Your sperm are the best!"
HOW YOU SAY IT: Delighted. Maternal.
RATIONALE: He'll be shocked at first, but pride will quickly become the overriding emotion.

WHAT YOU SAY: "Remember how we were trying to have a baby? Well . . ."

HOW YOU SAY IT: Reassuring. Maternal.

RATIONALE: He should be able to complete the sentence. If not, you may want to approach other candidates to fill the position of your baby's daddy.

WHAT YOU SAY: "What do you want for Father's Day?"

HOW YOU SAY IT: Supportive. Maternal.

RATIONALE: If you get a positive pregnancy result any time in the weeks leading up to the third Sunday in June, this may be a good option. Or at any other time really, presuming he has absolutely no idea when Father's Day is (seeing as you take care of all the card sending and other social niceties). It also implies that gifts will be coming his way.

WHAT YOU SAY: "I've got some news."

HOW YOU SAY IT: Somber. Maternal.

RATIONALE: This is a risky one. You want him to immediately feel worried that something awful has happened, so that when he finds out that it's only impending fatherhood he'll be pleasantly surprised and really quite relieved. Again, it's risky.

WHAT YOU SAY: "Look what I found in the bathroom!"

HOW YOU SAY IT: Confused. Maternal.

RATIONALE: For a few important seconds, you divert attention away from yourself and toward a positive pregnancy test wand. For a few important seconds, you and your partner are (ostensibly) united in shock and disbelief. This also gives your partner the opportunity to cleverly solve the apparent mystery, thus boosting his self-esteem and self-worth before he collapses on the sofa in shock.

If words completely fail you, you always have the option of simply silently brandishing the pregnancy test stick. This works only if it actually says the word "pregnant" in large uppercase letters. Do not expect a pattern of pink crosses and blue lines on a tiny piece of plastic held by a trembling hand to mean much to somebody on the brink of a life-changing, bank-account-ruining event.

STEP 3:
ARRANGE FOR BACKUP.

Beer tends to be the beverage of choice at times like these.

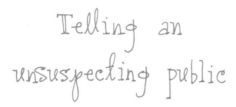

Telling an unsuspecting public

How to get the positive reaction you crave

If, in a feat of unprecedented restraint, you've managed to keep quiet about your conception efforts, you will have been lucky enough to avoid the incessant public commentary that inevitably accompanies an attempt at procreation—brilliant advice from the newly pregnant counterbalanced by dire warnings from the parents of two- and three-year olds. There is, however, one huge advantage in going public with your plans before they come to fruition—when you announce your pregnancy, everybody will know to be as thrilled and delighted as you are. But if you've played your hand close to your (lately blooming) chest, then your news may be met with less-than-enthusiastic reactions. These may include any of the following:

SURPRISE: "Wow! I didn't even know you were trying." (SUBTEXT: You simply can't imagine how pleased I am that this has happened to you and not to me.)

SYMPATHY: "Wow. I didn't even know you were trying."
(**SUBTEXT**: I don't want to be patronizing, but didn't I always say that something like this was going to happen?)

SHOCK: "What? I didn't even know you were trying!"
(**SUBTEXT**: I am shocked and appalled and can't wait to tell all of our mutual friends.)

STUNNED HORROR: "Whoa. I didn't even know you were trying."
(**SUBTEXT**: You two are *so* not ready to be parents.)

FEIGNED DELIGHT: "Wow!! I didn't even know you were trying!!"
(**SUBTEXT**: I'm feigning delight because I like to come across as a positive and upbeat person but frankly I'm horrified.)

Of course, the kind of reaction you get all depends on how you break the news. Saying simply "I'm pregnant" leaves your audience on the edge of a precipice, aware that one false verbal move could send them tumbling into the abyss of your ill humor. "Is this good news?" they ask themselves. "Is she to be congratulated or consoled?" "Does that wild-eyed expression on her face connote inexplicable joy or mind-numbing terror?"

Give your friends a sporting chance to stay on your holiday card list and prime them to give the response that you (in your newly fragile, hormonal state) desperately need. Precede your announcement with "I've got great news" or "Want to hear something really exciting?" These verbal cues will give them time to rearrange their features into the appropriate expression before the sheer magnitude of what you say wipes the smiles off their faces.

Even when you do lay the groundwork for a happy announcement joyfully received, there will always be some people who refuse to play along. For example:

PERPETRATOR: Your elder sister.

REACTION: Anger—she was planning on providing the first, and therefore most precious, grandchild.

REASON: She majored in Sibling Rivalry and wrote her thesis on Tattling and Subtle Pinching.

YOUR STRATEGY: Tell her that you just took a weekend course on Dirt-Dishing and will reveal to your parents exactly what she was doing, and who she was doing it with, that weekend she went on the tenth-grade retreat to knit blankets for Appalachian orphans.

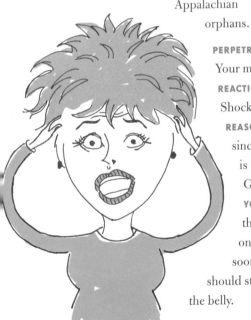

PERPETRATOR: Your mother.

REACTION: Shock.

REASON: Her greatest fear, since you first got your period, is of being addressed as Grandma.

YOUR STRATEGY: Tell her that if she ever wants to be on first-name terms with her soon-to-be grandchild, she should start out by being nice to the belly.

PERPETRATOR: Your immediate supervisor.

REACTION: Indifference, with just a hint of annoyance.

REASON: He sees his workload increasing exponentially as you spend the next six or seven months napping at your desk.

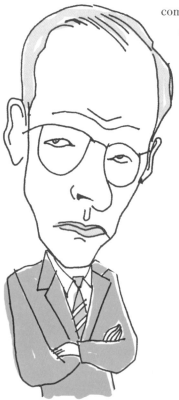

YOUR STRATEGY: Tell him that you are as committed as ever. Or tell him the truth, and say that you'll buy his lunch every day if he covers for you at your 9:00 A.M. status meetings.

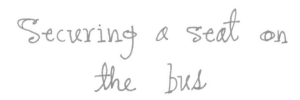
Securing a seat on the bus

How to appear more pregnant than you actually are

The second trimester is widely regarded as the halcyon days of a pregnancy. For the very first time in your life (it's fairly safe to assume), you are the proud owner of a small but unmistakable paunch. You have bundles of energy, a cheerfully hopeful disposition, and you're nausea free. You are not so enormous that you are perpetually uncomfortable. And the threat of childbirth is not so imminent that it washes over you in frequent, unbidden waves of horror, as if you had forgotten to study for your final exams or had hit *Reply All* when responding to a boss-bashing e-mail intended only for a like-minded colleague. Yes, the second trimester is pretty great.

Sad, then, that you are actually still in the first trimester. And it sucks. You feel sick, you're tired beyond belief, and you're a hormonal mess. This is the time when you need cartloads of support and kindness from your friends, your relatives, your coworkers, and, in a pinch, total strangers. Unfortunately, it's also the time when you look least pregnant and therefore are least likely to be the recipient of random acts of sympathy.

If you take public transport to work on a daily basis, or even if you deign to ride a bus or train only under extreme circumstances, you will know that as a pregnant commuter, your unwavering goal is to park your butt on a seat and keep it there while you fix your eyes on a point on the horizon and pray that you don't throw up. Feeling nauseous is bad enough, but feeling nauseous in a public place, squished up against sullen strangers in need of their morning caffeine fix, with no restroom, and nowhere to sit down for a three-mile, hour-and-fifteen-minute journey is surely every pregnant woman's ultimate nightmare.

Clearly, securing a seat is very, very important. But what do you do if, when you board your bus or train or whatever, all seats are selfishly occupied by nonpregnant and/or old people? You don't look pregnant, so no saintly soul is going to leap up and generously offer you his or her seat. (And, by the way, even when you do look pregnant, don't expect the great "I'm very absorbed in the business section of my newspaper" public to be particularly noble.) At this stage in the pregnancy game, you're contending with the "I'm not entirely sure you are pregnant and I don't want you to think that I think you're a bloater so I'll pretend that I'm very absorbed in the business section of my newspaper" public.

Ladies, you'll be delighted to hear that you have at your disposal a number of perfectly acceptable yet pleasingly cunning strategies, all designed to provide you with a prewarmed, vacant seat upon which you and your fetus may continue your journey in relative comfort:

CUNNING STRATEGY #1: *Look pregnant.* Simply stick your belly out. Even a first trimester tummy can take up room.

CUNNING STRATEGY #2: *Dress pregnant.* Empire waists exist for two reasons: To make very tall, very thin women look even more irritatingly gorgeous. And to make slightly nauseous, slightly chunky women like you look even more pregnant.

CUNNING STRATEGY #3: *Stand pregnant.* Place your hand in the small of back with your feet eighteen to twenty-four inches apart. Pregnant women don't actually stand like this, but you can assume that at least one seat hogger will be familiar with overly dramatic made-for-television movies and will quickly interpret your unusual stance as being that of a woman in the early stages of labor.

CUNNING STRATEGY #4: *Read pregnant.* Only the embryonically endowed read pregnancy books and magazines.

CUNNING STRATEGY #5: *Talk pregnant.* Call a friend on your cell phone and tell her (loudly) about your last prenatal appointment. Be sure to throw in words like *due date, ultrasound,* and (especially) *cervix.*

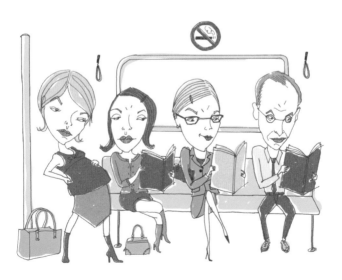

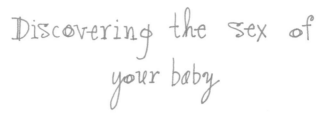

Discovering the sex of your baby

Why some secrets are best kept secret

Throughout your pregnancy people will ask you what
you're having, which is odd since it's presumably fairly
obvious that the answer is a baby. Depending on the
surroundings you may feel inclined to be facetious and say
"Ham and cheese on rye, please" or "Mine's a Guinness."
Take small pleasure in your own searing wit if you like,
but know that it's nothing more than a pointless avoidance
tactic. Accept the fact that for the next several months,
the boy or girl question will be the one most beloved of
strangers, bless their inquiring little minds. No doubt you
will reply (as your interrogator confidently expects) that
you really don't care if it's a boy or a girl as long as it's
healthy, and this is entirely true. Well, almost. The part
about wanting a healthy baby is true, but the part about
not caring what sex you have is just a big, fat fib.

Most people—most honest people, that is—if compelled to sit
down and have a really good think about it, would admit a preference
for one or the other. The reason is seldom deep and meaningful. You
may want a girl because the clothes are cuter or because you can't

think of any interesting boy names. Or a boy because *Little Man Tate* is your favorite film or because you'd like your partner to have someone to hang out with long term, thus freeing you up for a lifetime of spa facials and shopping trips. Whatever your inclination, it's all pretty much moot. Most of the time, you get what you're given, and the real issue is whether or not you should discover the sex of your offspring ahead of time.

If you're the kind of person who surreptitiously peels back the wrapping paper on gifts several weeks prior to December 25, or who simply can't wait the statutory ten minutes before pulling the little blackhead nabbing strip off your nose, expecting you to hang on for the better part of a year to learn the gender of your baby is simply cruel and unnatural torture. But if you possess a modicum of self-control, then please read on to see what you have to gain by not finding out. Or at least by not revealing your knowledge.

YOU'LL LEAVE YOURSELF WITH SOMETHING FANTASTIC TO LOOK FORWARD TO. Every twinge in the back, protruding hemorrhoid, and bout of flatulence confirms that you are, indeed, having a baby. Clearly, this is not news to you, or anybody else within a few feet of you, for that matter. Ah, but what kind of baby are you having? Will it be the son who excels in Little League? Or the daughter who flounces around the house in feather boas? Or even the son who flounces around the house in feather boas? There is no greater and more delightful surprise than discovering the sex of your baby. And there's no better time to do it than when that baby pops right out of you, and you can then say (at the risk of being mawkish), "Hi, little girl!" Or, "Boy, do you have big shoulders."

YOU'LL KEEP YOUR AUDIENCE IN A STATE OF HIGH ANTICIPATION. If people don't know what you're having, then the news that you've gone into labor, or that you're in the middle of pushing, or that you've actually had the baby, is of enormous interest to everyone. Suddenly, you and your baby are the hottest of topics. The excitement is palpable. What did they have? What did they have? they're all desperate to know.

When you've made the sex known beforehand, it all becomes a little humdrum. "Pass me the ketchup, and oh, did I tell you, Erin and Todd had their little boy," or "Before I forget, Aaron and Gina's daughter is here." The situation is even worse if you reveal both the sex and the name of your baby way before your due date. Then there's absolutely no whipping your public up into a frenzy of anticipation. It's all "Oh, by the way, Michael called to say that Hermione Jane arrived on Tuesday," which makes it sounds like she's coming home from college for the summer, rather than launching herself into the world after hiding incognito in the womb for nine months.

YOU'LL GIVE YOUR BABY MORE CLOTHING OPTIONS. When you've revealed the sex ahead of time, you'll be inundated with small garments in either pink or blue at your shower and other prebirth giving events. This is fine if you like pink or blue, but not knowing the sex of the baby forces people to be much more creative. You'll get lots of stuff in cream and yellow, green and orange, stripes and polka dots. Even if you hate orange, and pale green reminds you of that hideous bridesmaid dress they made you wear when you were twelve, you can't deny that your baby's first wardrobe will be much more interesting and colorful. Plus, in any case, after your baby is born, the same people will probably be generous enough to trot round with color-appropriate gifts to fill the small gaps in your child's already extensive closet.

YOU'LL AVOID JUMPING TO DANGEROUS CONCLUSIONS. Once you know the sex of your baby to be, you can pick out his or her name with absolute certainty. And from there, it's only a short hop, skip, and a jump to selecting your child's best subjects at school, the college he or she will attend, and how many people you're going to invite to the wedding reception. Well, not really, but you get the gist. Knowing that one critical fact about your baby predisposes you to making all kinds of other assumptions, when really you can know nothing about a person until you've actually met him or her. It also might cause you to name your baby—the child you confidently expect to be a mere slip of a girl, weighing about six pounds, with blue eyes and fair hair—something floral and feminine like Fay or Belle, when in fact you'll ultimately be giving birth to a chubby, red-faced howler who requires a name of an entirely different timbre.

Being demanding

Pregnancy is a fantastic excuse for pretty much anything.
Gaining weight? Check! Being bad tempered? Check!
Hitting the snooze button seven times in a row? Double
check! But why stop there? Why allow yourself these
minor social transgressions when, quite frankly, you can
get away with so much more? Remember, very few people
are brave enough to call out a pregnant woman, for fear
of the perceived consequences (which run the gamut
from tears to premature labor and often include sexual
harassment lawsuits and very public censure). This is one
of the few times in your life when you can be absolutely
true to the baser side of your nature with little fear of
retribution. Take time to explore—and enjoy—each of the
following Seven Acceptable Sins of Pregnancy:

1. **LAZINESS.** When it comes to domestic chores, you can most
definitely put your feet up, ideally while somebody else vacuums
the carpet under them. Nobody expects you to get down on
your hands and knees and scrub the bathroom floor when we
have it on good authority that inhaling the chemicals in cleaning
products means you'll have a two-headed kid.

2. BEING CONTROLLING. Having a baby is a really grown-up thing, which naturally means you should also take charge of lots of other smaller things. Consequently, you (and only you) operate the TV remote, decide how you're going to spend the weekend, and dictate where you all go for lunch. After all, somebody's got to make these decisions (and you're clearly the Person Most Likely to Have a Tantrum if Things Don't Go Her Way).

3. SELFISHNESS. When people believe that everything you do is in your baby's best interests, they'll overlook all kinds of petty behavior. So feel free to take the last doughnut. It's probably essential for fetal brain development or something.

4. UNPREDICTABLE CRYING. Everybody knows that pregnant women are highly emotional beings. You're simply at the mercy of all those hormones, so go ahead and bawl your eyes out whenever the mood strikes you. And if bawling gets you treats and sympathy, then so be it.

5. MAKING FOOD A PRIORITY. You're eating for two. You're nourishing a fetus. It helps keep your morning sickness at bay. You have to keep your energy level up. However you justify your obsession with food, it's all good.

6. TARDINESS. As you get bigger and bigger, it stands to reason that you're going to move slower and slower, and arrive later and later for every appointment and engagement. Never mind that you've never felt better, you're well hydrated, and you haven't had a hangover in months. As far as the great pregnancy-watching public goes, you operate at half speed. So enjoy the journey, rest awhile en route to that next meeting, and take as many snack breaks as you can afford.

7. **GETTING AWAY WITH MISTAKES.** Your brain is so full of new stuff (ostensibly preparing to be a parent, but in reality preparing to be a parent and making sure you have time to pick up ice cream on the way home from the office) that minor details like returning phone calls, collecting the dry cleaning, and actually going to work will inevitably slip through the cracks. It's just another fact of your glorious and self-indulgent pregnant life.

Giving the impression of relative normality

How to look pregnant without looking pregnant

One of the benefits associated with almost any change in personal circumstances (with the possible exception of a prison sentence) is the shopping. You graduate from college, and you simply must buy yourself a congratulatory gift. You get a new job, and you absolutely have to pick out a new wardrobe. You move into your first home, and it's basically required that you hang out in furniture stores, caressing sofas in an almost lascivious way.

Pregnancy is no exception. In fact, it's actually better, because it offers the double joy of shopping for a new baby (new furnishings, strange but fascinating pieces of equipment, darling little scraps of clothing) and for yourself (ditto, ditto, and ditto).

Of course, it hasn't always been this way. Society, and the mall, have not always been so kind to the givers of life. There was a time when, if a woman got in the family way, she'd suck it up, in, and any which way she possibly could in order to accommodate her growing girth within her existing wardrobe. She would go to any length (or width) to avoid (**A**) throwing down cash on a bunch of unsightly maternity dresses, and (**B**) actually wearing the aforementioned unsightly maternity dresses. When things got problematic, say around the fourth or fifth month, she'd grab her male companion's T-shirts, sweatshirts, and sweatpants, and with a deep and heartfelt sigh, commit to spending the last few months of her so-called confinement confined in fabric that would, in any case, soon be taut around the middle (although still very generously proportioned along the inseam and through the shoulders).

Times have changed and (sadly for anybody hoping to absorb the economic effects of pregnancy by giving up a magazine subscription or two) there are now many more options available to the fashion-conscious pregnant woman. In fact, with the notable exceptions of puffball skirts and leather bustiers, there are very few fashion trends that can't or haven't or shouldn't be adapted for a substantial belly simply by adding a little more fabric, with a little more give. Whatever your personal style, rest assured that you can hang onto it throughout your pregnancy.

This, of course, is very good news. As you slowly but surely lose control of the constants in your life, like your bra size and your bladder, it's nice to know that you don't have to wear those super-stretchy pants with an attractive inset belly panel (made of contrasting floral fabric) that come up to your armpits. Yes, you can still look young and trendy, even if you feel old and haggard. You can still sashay with a spring in your step. Actually, you can't because you're way too tired, but at least you can still look the part of girl-about-town (with a bun-in-the-oven).

These days, most maternity wear is designed to celebrate your new status as creator extraordinaire by showing off your growing bump in form-fitting styles. Along with paying homage to the immense change that's happening in your life, it also performs the useful function of assuring the world at large that, despite increasing evidence to the contrary, you are still the same person. And this is very important. As a pregnant woman you will be judged by your new appearance, and people will draw negative conclusions about your stamina and brain power simply because you are going to have a baby. Their flawed rationale is this: you are pregnant and therefore not committed to your job long term (you'll be going on maternity leave soon); not interested in your job (you probably spend all day shopping online for strollers); and incapable of actually doing your job (you're a veritable hormonal maelstrom and therefore an unpredictable presence in the workplace).

Maternity clothes that match your pre-pregnancy style and personality tell the world that it's still you under all that new padding. They say that you're still the same hard-working and committed member of the team or, alternatively, that you can still be relied on to sleep through most meetings and leave every day at four. The important message to all concerned is that yes, you happen to be having a baby, but otherwise it's business (or lack thereof) as usual.

Dressing for excess

Having accepted the fact that money will have to be spent on garments that you believe you only will wear for a few short months (based on the misguided notion that you'll actually have the time, the energy, and the inclination to go to the gym after the birth of your baby), it's important to assess the new body that you'll be dressing. As you know, Things Have Changed. Let's discuss:

BREASTS. If you're fairly flat chested by nature, it's almost worth getting pregnant simply for the novelty of having really big boobs for once in your life. But as is the case with all unexpected guests, there's the question of how, and where, to accommodate them. Think seriously about getting a couple of maternity bras. Not only are they bigger than your regular bras, but they're also constructed to offer more support, and as time goes by you'll be very glad they do.

BELLY. Make the most of your new asset by showing it off to maximum effect. Heck, you're pregnant—you might as well take advantage of it. Typically, the more pregnant you look, the more attention (admiring glances, comfy seats,

46

free food) you'll get from friends, coworkers, and even random strangers. To maximize this positive effect, it's possible, and even desirable, to flaunt the belly, depending on where you are and what you're doing. A day at the beach, sarong casually knotted below your bump? Absolutely. Big client presentation at work, sarong casually knotted below your bump? Probably not. The rules of appropriate dress are the same, pregnant or not, but as you get bigger you may find that the answers to your sartorial questions are quite literally beyond you.

At some point in your pregnancy, that cunningly constructed longer-in-the-front-but-still-tight-where-it-counts maternity T-shirt will start to resemble a was-I-drunk-when-I-bought-this? skimpy little top. Worse, *you may not even realize it.* This is because you may not actually be able to see over and beyond your belly and therefore have absolutely no idea what's happening on the underside of your curvature, where your shirt and your pants are in the process of an amicable but final divorce. New civilizations may have been discovered there, a Democratic president elected, inflation at a record low, but you wouldn't know. And while ignorance is generally blissful, for the sake of your coworkers of a nervous disposition, it's clearly time to invest in a full-length mirror.

BOTTOM. If your butt is expanding at about the same rate as your belly, you may think that heels are a good way to redress the balance. But *balance* is the operative word. No matter how much weight you think you've added to your rear end, it's never going to match what's happening out in front. Heels may make you more unsteady than ever on your feet, and taking a tumble when pregnant is neither safe nor particularly pretty. Plus, once you're down you may not be able to get up again without some assistance.

ANKLES. You expected to gain a belly, and maybe add a few inches to your chest, but the way your ankles inflate when you're pregnant is just beyond comprehension. Water retention plus gravity equals a tragic pair of pins. Pray that you're at the height of your pregnancy in the summer so that you can wear flip-flops with long, wide-legged pants or floor-skimming skirts, thus allowing your feet to breathe and the rest of us to be spared the awful truth. Try also to elevate your feet as much as possible. If you sit at a desk all day, think about fashioning a useful footstool from a discarded computer or plastic keg left over from last year's holiday party (which, by the way, is probably the last one you'll ever attend).

Defending the belly

How to preserve your personal space

Being pregnant means sharing your body with someone else. But voluntarily accommodating a baby is one thing; being subject to the hands-on approach of everyone you meet is quite another. For as soon as you are visibly with child, you will be touched, your belly rubbed, and your figure stared up and down. Previously pregnant women will check out your ankles (to see how swollen they are) and your bump (to see whether you're carrying high or low). The never-been-pregnant crowd will stare at your belly (because it's just so big and round) and your boobs (likewise). Maybe people think that because you were uninhibited enough to get pregnant in the first place you must have no concept of personal space. Or maybe people are just freaks.

Of course, it all depends on who's doing the touching. Close friends, your sister, even the father of your child may all be well within long-established rights to get intimate with your person. These are the people who hug and kiss you to say hello. They've seen you naked or, at the very least, wearing your oldest underwear. They can ruffle your hair, lean their head on your shoulder, pat you on the butt, and it's all just dandy. You know them and like them and feel comfortable with them in close proximity—and that's what sets them apart from the man standing next to you in line in the post office, the woman weighing your coffee beans, and the lady who shares your seat on the bus, all of whom feel an inexplicable need to connect on a tactile level with you and your lovely big belly.

The trick, then, is to create an impenetrable exclusion zone around your entire body and double layer it around the especially attractive magnet that is your tummy. Consider incorporating one or more of the following strategies into your personal armory:

DEVELOP AN UNAPPROACHABLE DEMEANOR. To a serious belly toucher, your bump just screams, "Caress me!" Be sure, then, that your face gives a stronger, contrary message—something along the lines of "Come any closer and I'll kick you really hard."

WEAR A LARGE HANDBAG DIAGONALLY ACROSS YOUR BODY. A really capacious purse acts like force field, protecting your belly from all comers. As a side benefit, it also means that you'll never be more than eighteen inches from your next snack. The only downside is that a purse slung across your middle, like horizontal stripes and pussycat bows, will only add to the illusion (or reality) of bulk.

RETCH SLIGHTLY, AS IF YOU MIGHT BE ABOUT TO THROW UP. For even the most ardent belly toucher, the unpleasant possibility of being vomited on outweighs the perceived pleasure of a good old pat.

SPELL IT OUT. Have a few T-shirts printed with a gentle and nonconfrontational message like "Hands off, lady" or "My body, my baby, my belly," or the modern classic, "I have Ebola."

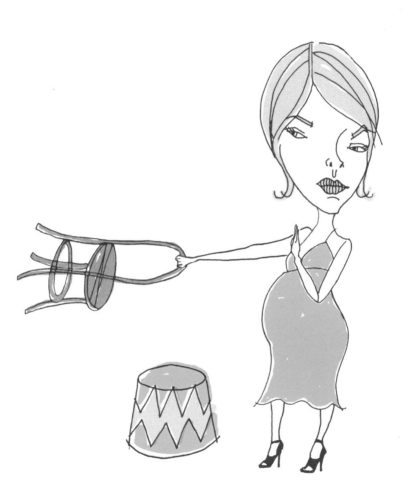

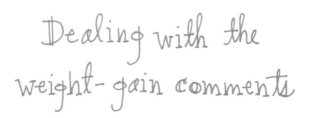

Dealing with the weight-gain comments

How to respond to so-called pregnancy humor

People are funny. They might say, "Cute haircut" or "I like your pants," but nobody's going to pat your love handles while remarking on the circumference of your midsection, or guffaw as they offer to make you a gag WIDE LOAD label to wear on the back of your coat. Not until you're pregnant, that is. Then, almost overnight, you become the butt, if you will, of everybody's attempts at the kind of humor that tries to be ingratiating but is mostly annoying.

The big problem with pregnancy humor is that it just isn't funny. Personal comments that poke fun at somebody's physical appearance usually aren't, and it seems doubly unfair to pick on a subsection of society that is (**A**) physically incapable of defending itself, being a little ungainly and all, and (**B**) in the throes of doing the very noble and admirable and underpaid job of becoming a mother.

Because internalizing all that negative karma is probably bad for your baby, be sure that you're ready with a choice retort for when the not-so-funny crowd descends. If you're the shy and retiring sort, pick from the top of the list, since they're somewhat gentler. If you have vicious heartburn and are feeling more than a little irritable, go straight to the last option, and enjoy yourself. But whatever you choose, never forget that you're pregnant. You're hormonal. You can get away with stuff like this.

THEM: "Wow! You're huge!"

YOU: "Oh, gosh, I love it. It's just so liberating not having to conform to society's idea of the perfect woman, for once."

RATIONALE: A mere suggestion of militant feminism can deter even the most resolute busybody.

THEM: "Wow! You're huge!"

YOU: "Do you think so? Really? Maybe I should stop eating so much."

RATIONALE: Ostensibly meek, this one will leave your tormentors backpeddling furiously, afraid that they have nudged you toward anorexia. If you've never allowed yourself the undeniable satisfaction of being passive-aggressive, this is a great way to start.

THEM: "Wow! You're huge!"

YOU: "Well, there's a baby in there. What did you expect?"

RATIONALE: You can laugh as you say this and it won't sound too harsh. But nobody will doubt what you mean. And how seriously you mean it.

THEM: "Wow! You're huge!"

YOU: "And you, too! What is it? Ten, twenty pounds?"

RATIONALE: Of course, this one works only if you know the person, but in the right circumstances it can be very powerful.

THEM: "Wow! You're huge!"

YOU: "Well, my hemorrhoids weigh a couple of pounds each."

RATIONALE: Any mention of an indelicate condition and vengeance is yours.

Breaking up with your doctor

What constitutes grounds for divorce

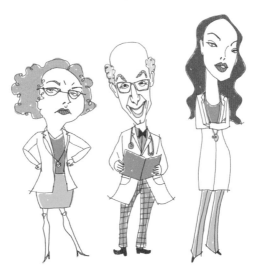

Before you got yourself in the family way, it's likely that the only personal contact you had with your gynecologist occurred annually and involved a cold metal speculum. Back then, even if you didn't really like him or her, you may have decided just to suck it up, so to speak, for those few minutes. But now that your pelvic region has an embryo in residence, two things change. Your gynecologist becomes your obstetrician. And you become worthy of closer and more frequent inspection.

Once you reach about eight weeks in your pregnancy, you'll see your doctor monthly until about week thirty-two, and then every two weeks until the last three weeks of your pregnancy. This makes for around twelve or thirteen visits, and more if your pregnancy is unusual in any way, so it's important that you actually like your obstetrician. Especially when you consider that he or she is the only person (other than you and the guy who donated his sperm) who has any real impact on the prebirth upbringing of your child. Granted, your body is already on a largely predetermined trajectory (destination: Toys 'R' Us), but your doctor can influence the course of your own little missile, particularly near the end of your pregnancy, when there are crucial decisions to be made about your labor (place of, duration of, and so on) and delivery (type of, narcotic availability during, that kind of thing).

Well before you get to that point (which, incidentally, is well beyond the point of no return), make sure that you and your doctor are of one mind on all the important stuff. Be on the lookout for doctor-patient disharmony in any of the following areas:

HIS OR HER MANNER. Why is it that when some people embark on a medical degree they are surprised to learn that their chosen profession requires them to interact with real people in a warm and fuzzy manner? While there are many, many kind-hearted, gentle-spirited doctors around, their number is matched by an equal number of cranky ones who treat questions with disdain and symptoms with disbelief. If your obstetrician apparently slept through Bedside Manner 101, then run as fast as your pregnant little legs will carry you. A gruff word to an overwrought pregnant woman can push her to the edge. And that's not a very comfortable place to birth a baby.

HIS OR HER ATTITUDE REGARDING WEIGHT GAIN. Some doctors adhere religiously to the unfair law of average pregnancy weight gain of between twenty-five and thirty-five pounds, with a little flexibility on either side if you start off very large or very small. On the other hand, some doctors (the nice ones) don't really care how much weight you put on as long as you eat right and stay healthy. If you find yourself gaining at an alarming rate at the beginning of your pregnancy (having fully embraced the wondrous if latterly discredited concept of eating for two), you may find yourself being chastised by your rail-thin female obstetrician. Or, worse, by your similarly svelte male practitioner.

HIS OR HER POSITION ON EPISIOTOMIES AND EPIDURALS. For you, some aspects of the whole birthing process might be complete and utter nonnegotiables. For example, you definitely don't want an episiotomy; you definitely do want an epidural. Or the other way around. (Or not.) These are very important issues. Find out where your doctor stands on them ahead of time, well before you are no longer in any position to protest.

HIS OR HER PERSONAL HYGIENE/TASTE IN SHOES/POLITICAL AFFILIATION. The pregnant woman is a highly sensitive being. Minor, inconsequential details that never caused a blip on your radar before pregnancy now become irritations the size of military jets. If your doctor's Southern accent, neighing laugh, or overuse of cologne gets on your nerves now, imagine how you're going to feel when you've been in labor for twenty-three hours. In reality, an annoying personal habit shouldn't be the reason you abandon a perfectly competent physician, but pregnancy is nothing if not a great excuse to be irrational.

If you believe that you have reason (however unreasonable) to leave your doctor, then you have two courses of action at your disposal:

FIND ANOTHER DOCTOR IN THE SAME PRACTICE. Even though your insurance company may have technically assigned you to one particular doctor, it may be entirely possible to see any of the other doctors in the practice at any prenatal visit. You may even be able to make a subtle, sideways, intrapractice doctor shift without anybody actually noticing.

COURT THE FAVOR OF A COMPLETELY NEW DOCTOR. Finding and wooing a doctor mid-pregnancy requires adherence to a special set of strategies, the details of which you will find upon turning the page.

Ingratiating yourself with a new doctor

How to present yourself as the perfect patient

Generally speaking, you don't have to pass an interview before a medical practice will accept you, assuming it is taking on new patients. But if you turn up at your first prenatal appointment seven and a half months pregnant, your new doctor may notice, and this astute medical observation may lead to some questions. You should, therefore, be prepared for what will feel (pregnant and sensitive as you are) like an interrogation.

Try to sound like a normal, sensible person as you elucidate why you left your last OB-GYN practice. Saying that you didn't like the color of the carpet in the waiting room or that the receptionist gave you funny looks is not really explanation enough, nor is it going to help you come across as the aforementioned rational person.

In anticipation of such an interview with your intended obstetrician, you are encouraged to work on at least one of the following excellent reasons for divorcing your former doctor:

SLIGHT MEDICAL INCOMPETENCE. Say something that hints at ineptitude, like the practice lost your records, or your doctor never had enough time to answer your questions. Because

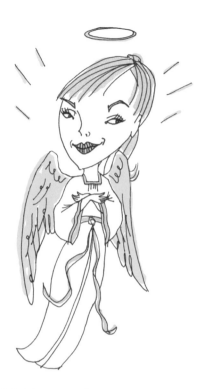

doctors are by definition overachievers, your new obstetrician will delight in immediately proving him- or herself better than your former practitioner. It's to your advantage to foster this healthy competition.

INCONVENIENT LOCATION. Say that because of the increasing frequency of your prenatal visits, you need a doctor closer to your place of work than to your home. This will make you seem like an efficient, punctual, no-nonsense kind of gal. It gives the impression that you will arrive at appointments on time, ask a minimum of questions, and, best of all, have all your insurance paperwork complete and up-to-date. The practice receptionist will adore you.

DIFFERENCE OF OPINION. Subtly give the impression that your old doctor is a sadistic maniac who performs episiotomies for fun and delights in denying drugs to laboring women. (Try not to use words like *sadistic* and *maniac,* since this will only make you seem more hormonally challenged than you actually are.)

When you've convinced your obstetrician-to-be that you were justified in leaving the last practice, you need to present yourself as a patient who will really add value to the new one. Thanks to the Internet and the Discovery Health Channel, you probably know more about your unborn child than your new doctor does. Keep this fact to yourself. Try to appear a little clueless, but not so dumb ("So you're saying that I should quit smoking?") that you're a medical liability. On the other hand, you don't want to come across as a smart-ass know-it-all ("Remind me, doctor, is my placenta anterior or posterior?"). It's important that you make your doctor feel truly needed, as if all that time and money invested in medical school were leading up to this one, hugely satisfying appointment.

Once you've been accepted by your new doctor, don't rest on your laurels. You've done a fine job of convincing everyone that you're about as unhormonal as a pregnant woman can safely be, but you have weeks, maybe even months, ahead of you during which you must maintain a strong and mutually beneficial relationship with your new doctor and his or her cohorts. Try to follow these simple rules:

MAKE NICE WITH THE RECEPTIONIST. This is the person who holds sway over the coveted first-thing-in-the-morning or last-one-of-the-day appointment. You need him or her on your side at all times.

ARRIVE ON TIME FOR YOUR APPOINTMENT. Don't assume that your doctor will run behind every time, just because he or she has run behind every time *so far*. This is a very dangerous mistake to make (dangerous in the sense that it won't leave you with enough time in the waiting room to peruse, and possibly borrow, your favorite magazines).

DON'T COMPLAIN WHEN YOUR DOCTOR'S RUNNING LATE. It's probably because he or she has been delivering a baby. Think about it—you'd probably rather your doctor sticks around for the last fifteen minutes of your labor instead of scurrying back to the office for some neurotic woman's five-month visit.

DON'T COMPLAIN ABOUT THE AMOUNT OF WEIGHT YOU'VE GAINED. Compared with his or her patients with preterm labor, gestational diabetes, or triplets, the extra few pounds that have mysteriously attached themselves to your butt will be of little medical interest to your doctor.

DON'T ASK FOR A REWEIGH. Those expensive hospital-grade scales never lie.

DON'T COMPLAIN ABOUT STRETCH MARKS. You'll either get them or you won't. And if you do, your doctor can't help you. And if he's a man, he won't care anyway.

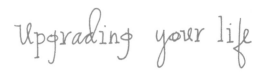

Upgrading your life

How to use your pregnancy for personal enrichment

Even if having a baby is the fulfillment of all your hopes and dreams, there's no denying that it involves some pretty significant lifestyle changes, not all of them positive. For a start, everything is more expensive—you've invested in a whole new wardrobe to accommodate your new shape; you go to the bathroom at least ten times more often every day and toilet paper isn't cheap; and you feel compelled to buy every pregnancy book out there, just in case one of them has the secret to a short and painless labor.

And it's true: pregnancy isn't always a lot of fun. In your less nauseated moments, you'll probably miss your previous extravagant social life. Now, a wild night to you means an extra half hour in front of the TV and marshmallows on your cocoa. Nobody relishes the prospect of waking up with the fullest bladder in the known universe, or going to bed with heartburn and one of those ridiculously large comforter-hogging body pillows.

To counteract the pitfalls of pregnancy, allow yourself the pleasure of maximizing its perks and make a concerted effort to upgrade your life wherever and whenever possible. It is commonly held that you are well within your rights as a pregnant person to utilize your new status in order to do the following:

PREBOARD ON PLANES. It's not good for you to stand around for long periods of time, especially when you're surrounded by irritating people with too much carry-on baggage. Tell the gate stewards that you're pregnant (but not so pregnant that you're a liability) and that you really need to sit down (preferably in business class) or else you might faint (loudly and with scant regard for other passengers). With any luck, this will also net you preferential in-flight treatment (like an extra bag of pretzels or more than one ice cube).

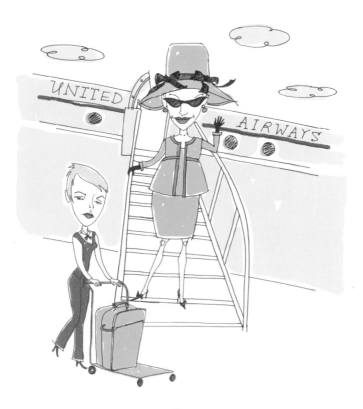

GET THE BEST TABLE AT YOUR FAVORITE RESTAURANT. You're pregnant, so you're probably really aware of things that just don't bother less-productive people. You're very sensitive to lighting and noise, and you have just realized that feng shui makes a huge difference in controlling your heart palpitations. That cute corner banquette with all the candles will probably do.

REWARD YOURSELF WITH AN OCEAN VIEW. Hotel staff are always looking for reasons to upgrade people to the really nice rooms that nobody can afford anyway. Pregnancy is a perfect pretext, so you'll actually be doing them a favor by laying it on thick. Tell them it's your last weekend away with your partner before the baby is born. Recount some tale of woe in which you lose your job, or the paint in the nursery turns out to be a horrid acid green rather than the soft buttery yellow you'd hoped for. Say that pregnancy has brought on your latent claustrophobia, and if they can give you anything bigger (preferably a penthouse suite), then everybody's life is going to be considerably more pleasant.

CUT IN LINE AT THE GROCERY STORE. Next to standing around at Gate 19B, standing around at the supermarket checkout may be the worst kind of standing around for pregnant women to do. (And don't even think about standing around at the DMV.) Until there's a checkout reserved specifically for pregnant women, you have every right to take yourself to the head of the line, murmuring soft little apologies while making sure that your poor, distended belly bumps against everybody's shopping cart.

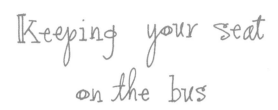

Keeping your seat on the bus

How to appear more pathetic than you actually are

It's the tail end of your second trimester and you are just blooming. Words like *fulsome* and *burgeoning* were invented for the exact purpose of describing you (along with *massive, unwieldy,* and *rotund*). You're simply bursting with baby, bonhomie, and the carefree attitude of someone who thinks she's soon to leave the drudgery of the nine to five to cavort happily with a small, sweet friend (little realizing that the daily grind is about to become the nightly turmoil).

But aside from the fact that you and your belly are about as perfect and happy a couple as any that have waddled this earth, there's absolutely no reason why you should experience any shortfall in public sympathy. This is most definitely the time to exploit your obvious size and mobility issues. So remember, a seat on a bus is yours by right, and your extreme vitality should in no way stand between you and a pernicious octogenarian. Work on appearing pathetic and exhausted, and do nothing to make yourself look perkier than you actually are. Hair and makeup should be attended to only *after* you've reached your destination, or not at all. For maximum effect, try to follow these additional guidelines:

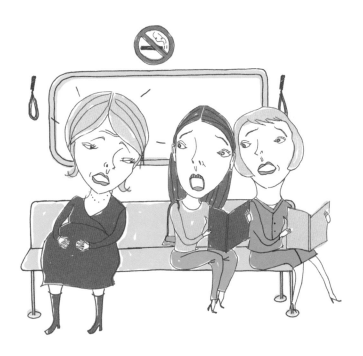

NEVER TRY TO DISGUISE YOUR BUMP. By now it's probably reaching embarrassing proportions, and in order to stave off horrified looks you might feel compelled to hide it a little. Don't even try—just be proud of that prize-winning pumpkin of yours, and use it to your advantage.

CAPITALIZE ON THE FACT THAT MOST PEOPLE ARE MORTALLY AFRAID OF HAVING TO STEP UP IN A CRISIS. People can be just plain selfish—they'll do anything not have to deliver a baby on their way to work. You don't have to overdo it, but anything that might suggest that your baby's head is crowning right then and there can only further your cause. Belly clutching is useful, as is the occasional wince.

SHOW OFF THOSE CHUNKY LITTLE ANKLES OF YOURS. Water retention is pretty much a fact of life as your pregnancy progresses, but they (the evil seat hoarders) needn't know it. If your ankles and/or calves are horrendous to behold, don't hide them. And if you need any justification for swindling some poor senior out of her seat, know that standing while in transit will only exacerbate your edema. (And edema trumps emphysema every time.)

STAND CLOSE TO A SEATED PASSENGER WHILE HOLDING (AT HIS EYE LEVEL) WHAT SEEMS TO BE A URINE SAMPLE. Plus, when you get off the bus you'll have a nice, refreshing apple juice to tide you over as you amble to your destination.

Furnishing the perfect nursery

How to finagle a lucrative baby shower

Until about the age of two, your baby won't know that he's sleeping in a shallow cardboard box that once held a dozen six-packs, upon a mattress cleverly fashioned from an old pillowcase stuffed with discarded hosiery. Yet from the time of conception until the moment of birth, his needs— real or imagined—grow exponentially. And expensively.

As you have certainly discovered by now, part of the fun of having a baby is the shopping. But even more fun than the shopping is having someone else pick up the tab. Fortunately, this is exactly what baby showers are for. Sure, they're a great opportunity to congratulate you on your impending motherhood, gather your girlfriends together, and drop cake crumbs on someone else's rugs, but they're also possibly the only way that your baby is going to enter the world and find it fully equipped with everything he needs, and a lot of things he doesn't.

The other great reason for having a baby shower is to make sure that you don't end up spending all your much-needed postpartum cash on someone who, quite frankly, doesn't care whether his top matches his pants. Or even whether he's wearing pants. Ensure that your own baby shower delivers by simply following these strategies:

MAKE A LIST. Go window shopping, research online, read product reviews, and figure out *exactly* what you want—what brand, size, color, and quantity—and then make a very detailed list. Remember, this is not the time to be vague. If you are anything less than absolutely specific when asked the question "Is there anything you need?" you can bet your bottom dollar (the one which will then have to be spent on clothing your new child) that you will get things you don't like or already have.

REGISTER. Scribbling things down on a scrap of paper may make you feel better (less mercenary) than compiling a registry at a store or online, but a list's a list. The only difference is that when you register officially, your illegible handwriting won't cause you to end up with two diaper bags when really you meant two packages of cloth diapers.

DON'T BE GREEDY. Go for small-ticket items. A humble pack of washcloths, a bottle of baby shampoo, a nail clipper—it's all good. And it's all money that you don't have to spend on the baby equivalent of an oil change, or toilet paper, or some similarly tedious but necessary purchase. The less of the regular, everyday, boring stuff you have to buy yourself (diapers, for example), the more cash you'll have to spend on yourself and your postpartum comforts.

DON'T BE SELF-EFFACING. Maybe one person by herself won't spring for that fabulous stroller that all the celebs have, but people are pack animals and they like to give in groups. So if you really want it, really ask for it.

AVOID THE UNNECESSARY. This is a great time to talk to other moms and get their advice about what you do and don't need.

For example, the books may tell you to purchase twelve small, kimono-style undershirts for the first month of your baby's life (**A**) so that you need to do laundry only once a day, and (**B**) because a nasty old onesie might rub against your infant's delicate cord stump and break it off prematurely (and messily). However, the truth is that a loose onesie is perfectly fine, that yucky stuff gets everywhere anyway, and that cord stumps are tougher than you think. Before you make your final decisions, remember to talk to a new mom who's on your wavelength. Don't ask your cousin who has elevated neuroticism into an art form unless, of course, you're even more neurotic. In which case you've already purchased, washed, ironed, and put away your twelve small, kimono-style undershirts.

DON'T ASK FOR THINGS YOU CAN LIBERATE FROM THE HOSPITAL YOURSELF. A bulb aspirator (a.k.a. snot snatcher) is a good example. On leaving the hospital a day or two after your baby's birth, you'll be able to walk away (albeit uncomfortably) with at least one, as well as a handful of digital thermometers.

DON'T UNDERESTIMATE HOW FAST BABIES GROW. Or even how big they can be when they come out. Apparently, the average baby weighs about seven and a half pounds. Which means that in order for some babies to be average, there must be non-average babies on either end of the weight chart—delicate little slips of things around the five-pound mark, and great, hefty ten-pounders. Both extremes are fine, both can be perfectly healthy, and both can completely screw up your well-laid plans. So ask for things in a variety of sizes—bigger rather than smaller—and take into account the time of year when your baby will be born. Nobody wants to wear angora in August.

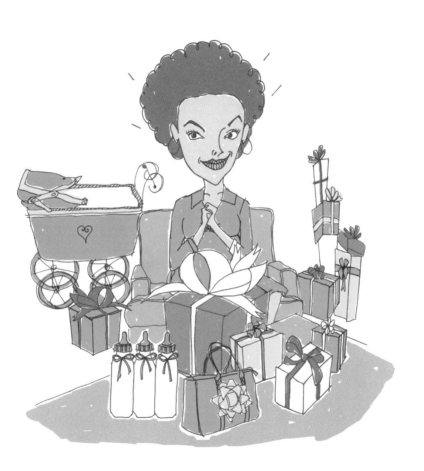

Naming your child

Probably the most exciting thing about having a child—for other people, at least—is naming it. You've confirmed, by creating a baby, that you're a superior being, and now everybody hopes you'll take yourself down a peg or two by giving it a terrible moniker.

As you may already have discovered, all the people you know (and some you don't) have a point of view on the subject of suitable and appropriate names for your child. Which is why, from the moment you announce your pregnancy, you can confidently expect one of three things to happen:

SCENARIO 1:

People will ask you whether you've thought of any names. You'll tell them the ones you're thinking of. Then they'll have an opinion (usually contrary to yours because there's really no fun in agreeing), which they'll share with you.

SCENARIO 2:

People will ask you whether you've thought of any names. You'll tell them the ones you're thinking of. Then they'll have an opinion, but they'll keep it to themselves. Subsequently, they'll persist in referring to your unborn by the name you casually threw out as a front-runner in week twenty-three of your pregnancy (but grew to loathe by week twenty-five).

People will ask you whether you've thought of any names. You'll say no.

The main advantage of this last scenario is that it keeps contentious conversation to a minimum. You won't have to fend off unwanted opinions when you simply don't have the energy or the inclination to fight for your right to dig *Ernestina* out of obscurity, or to explain why naming your child *Horatio* or *Napoleon* is simply an expression of your child's presumed uniqueness and individuality, and not a cross he'll have to bear for the rest of his life.

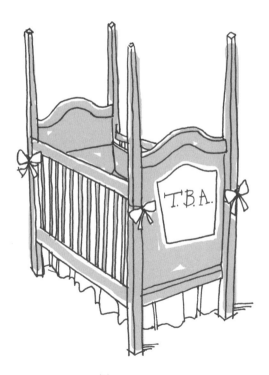

Keeping mum from the get-go also gives you an almost infinite window of opportunity (limited only by the arrival of your baby) to read up on names, research naming strategies, formulate your own shortlist, and—most important—adopt at least one of the following excellent and immutable reasons for ensuring that you (to the exclusion of everyone else around you, including, of course, the father-to-be) get the last word:

ESTABLISH YOUR NAMING STYLE AS PREEMINENT. A lot of naming indecision (and, consequently, unfortunate decision making) comes about because of the different naming styles of the two parents. Pregnancy tends not to resolve this issue, as the combination of overtired and high-strung mother-to-be and crabby and in-denial father-to-be often makes a mutually agreeable decision even more elusive.

Under these circumstances, your best plan is to establish irrefutable grounds for why your naming style is the gold standard. Point to the row of baby-naming books on your bookshelf, or the reams of articles you've downloaded from the Internet. Quote statistics—the popularity of certain names by year or state, the relative scholastic successes of *Mildreds* and *Madeleines.* Treat the whole matter as a scientific subject worthy of much research and reflection—somewhat akin to choosing one's fantasy baseball team, for example—and one that demands an expert adjudicator (you).

MAKE A DETAILED LIST. Instead of having a bunch of names floating around in your mushy pregnant brain, write them down on a piece of paper. Be sure to compose your list using only those names that you would actually consider naming your child, not those that you think sound cool when applied to the children of movie stars (nouns related to fruit, geography, and musical instruments tend to fall into this category).

The other great advantage of making a list is that there's something official about having things down on paper. When your partner offers some random eleventh-hour suggestion of his own, you can simply reply, "Hmm. Let me check. No, sorry, it's not on The List." Be sure to carry The List with you at all times. You're pregnant, so you know that your short-term memory is nothing but a memory. Things will get better after you have your baby (better for your brain, at least), but in the meantime, you'll want to be sure you have The List on hand at all times, just in case.

Eloise
Giselle
Portia
Sabine
Bailey

PICK YOUR MOMENT. If you suspect that your partner may be unwilling to give up his own favorites, however hideous and inappropriate they may be, bide your time and keep your opinions to yourself. Instead of spending six or seven weeks debating the relative merits of *Brittney, Brittany, Brittuny,* and *Brittanee,* work on developing an aura of calm compliance as you wait for the perfect moment, which usually reveals itself when you are in the throes of labor, coiled up in pain, sweaty and desperate. Your partner, if he's a remotely decent chap, will find it hard to refuse you anything as you strain and struggle to perpetuate his genes.

However you get appointed (or appoint yourself) to the position of Chief Namer, be sure that you (the singular *you,* that is) have made your decision some time before your baby is born, as wrestling with the vagaries of a newborn may cloud your otherwise excellent judgment. All too frequently, new parents seem to (**A**) make a hasty naming decision when presented with a swaddled infant, or, more commonly, (**B**) make a hasty naming decision when presented with a swaddled infant while still under the influence of childbirth-related drugs (her) or childbirth-related alcohol (him). There is a reason why numerous children end up with names like *Amnesia, Nocturne,* and *Glory.* And don't forget, if you complete the appropriate birth registration forms with your baby's name while you're in the hospital they'll actually submit the paperwork for you. To someone who's still figuring out how to unsnap a nursing bra, this will be a very appealing offer.

Remember, naming your baby is definitely one of the perks of the whole experience. It's a challenge, to be sure, a responsibility even, but after all the doctor visits, the prodding and the poking, the self-denial, and the abstinence, naming a baby can be the most fun and creative part of the whole experience (barring the initial fun and creative part).

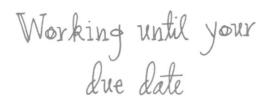

Working until your due date

How to get paid for being pregnant

If you're feeling slightly resentful that they still force you to sit at a desk all day when all you want to do is collapse on the sofa, watch daytime TV, and eat bon-bons, then here's a little mind game that you can play with yourself: pretend that instead of doing whatever you're supposed to do at work, your real job is to have a baby, and that everything you do from nine to five (or ten to three-thirty, depending on how conscientious you are) is done with the single-minded goal of furthering your very successful career as Senior Pregnant Person. You'll soon find that the workplace offers many opportunities for perfecting your pregnancy skills, and it's simply up to you and your fetus to take advantage of them. Make sure your schedule includes the following:

FREE BOTTLED WATER. If drinking the recommended eight glasses of water every day is a chore, you'll delight in how much easier it becomes when somebody else is paying for it. Plus there's the added bonus of being able to while away a good chunk of your day around the water cooler discussing TV's latest foray into soft porn with your fellow slackers.

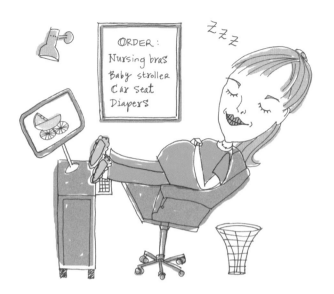

ORDER:
Nursing bras
Baby stroller
Car seat
Diapers

PAID NAP TIME. If you work in anything close to a corporate environment, you probably have a computer monitor on your desk. And a monitor on your desk usually means some kind of computer-like box thing under your desk. And it's funny, isn't it, how often you have to reboot the thing. And how difficult it is to find that minuscule reboot button. And how, when you're down there searching for it, being the technically minded and proactive person you are, you just happen to put your head down and close your eyes for a minute or two.

NO-CHARGE INTERNET ACCESS. Find answers to those burning pregnancy questions—"If I eat three bars of chocolate a day, will I exceed my daily caffeine allowance? Do I need to take a bathrobe to the hospital or will modesty simply not be an option at that point?" — that just can't wait until your next doctor visit. And what better way to do your research than on the Internet, while ostensibly investigating the economic effects of the health care crisis or looking up the dictionary definitions of *discrete* and *discreet*. Plus, it means that you won't be constantly on the phone to your doctor's office, so you're actually saving your employer time and money.

PHONE CALLS ON THE HOUSE. Talking of which, because your clients (doctors, hospitals, insurance companies) and your vendors (crib emporiums, baby clothing stores, diaper services) keep regular business hours, you have no choice but to use the phone on your desk for coordinating all your pregnancy projects.

GRATIS OFFICE SUPPLIES. Sometimes it's good to take a break from the same old routine and free your mind by doing something more creative, like selecting envelopes for your baby's birth announcements from the stationery cupboard. You'll probably return to your original task so much fresher and generally more inspired.

COMPLIMENTARY SNACKS. To maintain your energy level at a constant, sugar-induced high, enjoy the boost that only free workplace food can provide. Leftovers from a client lunch (look for high-protein sandwiches, fruit salads, and oatmeal cookies) complement the regular fare of Monday's bagels and Friday's doughnuts. If you're really smart, you'll figure out a way to rig the vending machine so that you can get a candy bar for a nickel.

FEE-FREE ADVICE. The whole maternity leave and insurance claims thing can be a bit daunting. Fortunately, you have at your disposal a lovely human resources person whose job description compels him or her to give you endless smiling advice, just when he or she would really rather be sorting out the screwup in payroll. Be sure to pop by regularly.

Visiting the beauty Salon with just days to go

How to rationalize that last-minute appointment

Whatever your choice of birthing environment, you will, no doubt, have ensured that your child is greeted by a team of professionals experienced in the art of baby catching and located in relatively sanitary surroundings. So far, so good. The world, to your newborn, seems populated by mature and sensible grown-ups, sporting clean clothes and fairly tidy hair. But what of you, her mother? From whatever exit route she emerges, the chances are that her all-important, relationship-defining first impression of you will be determined solely by your heinous six-month-old pedicure. Shrieking of lack of attention to detail and dubious personal hygiene standards, it also 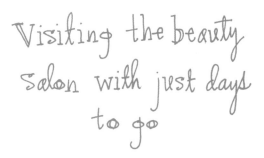 strongly suggests that you are destined to be the kind of mother who is blind to a snotty nose of tidal wave proportions and who restricts all that fun bath time stuff to a paltry once-a-week event.

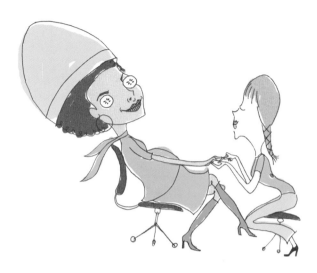

And creating a positive first impression isn't the only perfectly sound reason for rescheduling your thirty-eight-week doctor visit so you can get the appointment that just opened up with your favorite aesthetician. Read on for more ways to justify your last-minute spa treatment.

IT COULD BE A LONG, LONG, LONG TIME BEFORE YOUR NEXT VISIT TO THE BEAUTY SALON. The first few weeks after the birth of your baby will be a merry dance of feeding, changing, and sleeping (but not for you). If you can't find time to have a morning shower, there's little hope for highlights and a manicure. So do it now, before your baby's born. In fact, do every useful, practical, or edifying activity that you possibly can ahead of time. This includes sleeping and eating.

THINK OF THOSE FIRST MOTHER-AND-BABY PHOTOS. Hair plastered across your sweaty forehead and mascara settling on your cheekbones may stand as testimony to the effort you've gone through to push that reluctant baby into the world. But a brow wax and a facial is going to look so much better in the album.

YOU SIMPLY DESERVE IT. If you've been working throughout your pregnancy, be sure to give yourself a few days of vacation time before your due date and spend them being pampered. Don't fall into the silly trap of hoarding up all your precious leave time just so you can spend every last minute of it with your progeny. While it's an admirable notion in theory, remember that in the relaxed and soporific atmosphere of the spa it's way easier to attend to a demanding baby via your terribly handy umbilical cord.

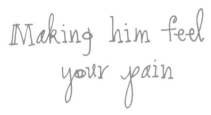

Making him feel your pain

How to share your pregnancy symptoms with the father-to-be

At this point, you've undoubtedly forgotten that making a baby was a joint decision, one that you both entered into with your eyes wide open and your eager, innocent hearts full of joy. Right now, your mutual pregnancy seems about as much of a partnership as it would if *you* were out scaling Everest while *he* relaxed at the base camp in front of a roaring fire, cradling a steaming chalice of mulled wine. You're suffering from heartburn, hemorrhoids, water retention, and a severely compromised mood; his life remains relatively unchanged.

Which is why it's about time your partner got a little closer to the whole experience. And we're not talking about making him wear one of those thirty-pound strap-on bellies, despite the high amusement value. Instead, start thinking of small but meaningful ways to introduce your partner to the highlights of pregnancy on a more personal level.

This strategy offers you two undeniable benefits: You'll feel better about your own discomfort watching your partner suffer. And thinking up new tortures will take your mind off your own terrible indigestion or whatever it is that occupies your every waking (or sleeping) hour.

YOUR PHYSICAL SYMPTOM:
BACKACHE

HOW TO HELP HIM EXPERIENCE IT: Have him rearrange the furniture in every room of your home several times, using your soon-to-arrive offspring as the pretext. Living room seating should be positioned just so, allowing you to watch TV or look out of the window while you're nursing. The baby's room should be organized so that everything is within an arm's reach of the changing table, with no more than one piece of furniture placed along any single wall. And your antique cast-iron claw-foot bathtub would work so much better three inches to the left. Be sure to sit in the most comfortable chair while directing the maneuvers, and then change your mind and have him go through the whole tortuous process again.

YOUR PHYSICAL SYMPTOM:
INSOMNIA

HOW TO HELP HIM EXPERIENCE IT: Useful nighttime tactics include tossing and turning relentlessly; switching the light on and grumbling loudly every time you get up to pee; and asking to change sides of the bed on the hour, every hour, because you just can't seem to get comfy where you are. You should also make him join you in consuming the recommended sixty-four fluid ounces of water every day. In addition to necessitating frequent nightly trips to the bathroom, this will also help him feel *bloated*.

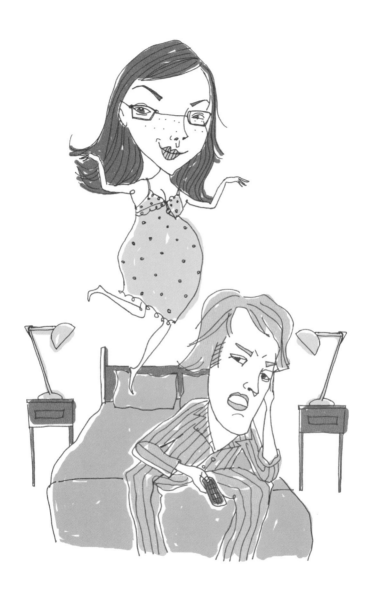

YOUR PHYSICAL SYMPTOM:
HEARTBURN

HOW TO HELP HIM EXPERIENCE IT: Insist on cooking for him—say that you find it therapeutic, now that your morning sickness has subsided, and that you're planning on trying out lots of fun and interesting recipes from your brand-new cookbooks (*Spice It Up!* and *Not for the Lactose Intolerant!*). Tragically, owing to an unspecified pregnancy-related condition, you will be unable to sample the fruits of your labors yourself, of course. If you are an extremely bad cook, you may strike it lucky and be able to add *nausea* to his repertoire of new pregnancy symptoms.

YOUR EMOTIONAL SYMPTOM:
IRRITATION

HOW TO HELP HIM EXPERIENCE IT: Make sure that you lose the TV remote when his favorite program is on, so he'll be compelled to sit through another one of those renovating-your-home-with-no-money-and-even-less-taste shows that he hates.

YOUR EMOTIONAL SYMPTOM:
FORGETFULNESS

HOW TO HELP HIM EXPERIENCE IT: Send him on long and complicated missions to the grocery store or the pharmacy for items that you absolutely cannot live without. When he returns, chastise him for forgetting something that you never asked him to get in the first place. As well as making him experience the misery of sudden-onset forgetfulness, it will add to his overwhelming sense of *irritation* (see above).

YOUR EMOTIONAL SYMPTOM: *WEEPINESS*

HOW TO HELP HIM EXPERIENCE IT: Consistently reveal the final scores of all the ball games he has to tape while he's repainting the baby's room for the third or fourth time. This may also lead to *extreme anger,* although that is not, strictly speaking, a symptom of pregnancy.

Requesting hospital-grade narcotics

How to pitch the question successfully

In all the flurry of getting pregnant, picking out maternity wear, and buying baby clothes, it may have escaped your attention that, at some point, you'll likely have to experience a degree of pain in order to release your progeny into the world. So as you approach the Big Day, take a moment or two to consider the notion that having a baby can hurt a bit, and ponder possible options for relieving said discomfort.

With their due dates in sight, most heavily pregnant women fall into one of two camps. Either they're of the mind that pain can be managed by performing breathing exercises, or by self-hypnosis, or by some other noninvasive means, and that childbirth is actually a very powerful and emotionally gratifying experience. Or they're of the mind that pain sucks, even if you get something really nice at the end of it, and if someone's offering you drugs it's just plain rude to refuse them.

Drugs, of course, aren't the only option, but the thing about drugs—as opposed to breathing, visualization exercises, and self-hypnosis—is that using them to your advantage relies entirely on the willing cooperation of another person, typically somebody with some background in the medical profession. Unfortunately for you, this means that the person choosing your pain management method is someone who (extensive viewing of *ER* reveals) (**A**) works fifty-eight-hour shifts and lives on black coffee, doughnuts, and premade sandwiches, and (**B**) spends his or her days stitching up people whose arms are hanging off or who have nails embedded in their skulls. As a result, that person's threshold for tolerating (someone else's) pain tends to be high. While calmness in the face of crisis is to be applauded, a pedestrian tempo ("Let's just complete the last of your insurance forms before we do anything else, shall we?") may be very bad news for you and your sudden need for narcotics.

Getting the message across that you really, *really* need something to take the edge off the pain is all a question of strategy. Formulate yours before your decision-making powers become a thing of the past (usually somewhere between five and ten centimeters). Consider the following:

> **FIRST, DECIDE WHERE YOU STAND ON THE ISSUE.** There are some very good reasons not to take drugs. On this, one of the most important days (or nights) of your life, wouldn't it be nice to experience it with your senses intact and your head as clear as a bell? After all, it's not a frat party or a blind date or some such occasion when you pray for post-event amnesia. Plus, as you know, whatever goes into your body also ends up, by the miracle

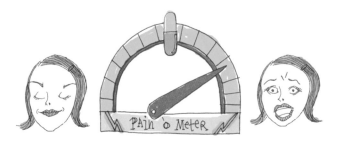

of the umbilical cord and the placenta, in your baby's body. This applies as much to hospital-administered narcotics as it does to second-hand smoke and tequila shots. Which means that while drugs may afford you some relief, they may also make your newborn pretty sleepy for the first day or so of his or her life in the big world. Normally, successfully combining the words *sleepy* and *newborn* in the same sentence would be cause for celebration, but a tired newbie isn't exactly what you need when you're trying to get the hang of breastfeeding and one participant just (yawn) can't (yawn) be bothered (yawn).

On the other hand, there's something to be said for not being so consumed by the pain that your memory of the whole birthing event forever has touches of the macabre about it. Maybe you don't want to win the prize for Most Awful/Dramatic/Surreal Childbirth Experience in your mothers' group. The bottom line— have an idea about where you stand on the epidural question. And even if you think you've made a decision one way or the other, make sure everyone knows that you reserve the right to change your mind (at any time and about anything, really).

SECOND, BE WILLING TO SHOW YOUR EMOTIONS. If you are able to be calm and polite as you make your request, your need may not seem so pressing to those in charge of the pain-relief meds. To get your point across, consider bawling and/or screaming in the delivery room. And if you *really* need an epidural, this is probably what you are already doing.

THIRD, SAY THANK YOU NICELY. Within minutes of receiving an epidural, you will undergo the most rapid mental and physical transformation of your entire life. You'll move from horror and panic—the kind that's typically associated with the sensation of having a bowel movement about the size of that birthing ball you never got to use—all the way across the emotional spectrum to a lovely, squishy, fluffy feeling of total and utter relaxation, albeit tinged with the kind of reckless abandonment that makes you overlook the fact that your bare bottom is hanging out of your hospital gown. You'll notice (and probably even feel inclined to point out in a giggly fashion) what a terribly attractive man (or woman) the anesthesiologist is. You'll even start joking with the doctor stationed between your legs. You'll check out your surroundings, maybe watch a little TV. You'll gently chastise your partner for forgetting the video camera (or for remembering the video camera). The whole occasion will start to assume the air of a jolly nice cocktail party, where everybody hangs around making casual conversation, nibbling on hors d'oeuvres, and enjoying expertly mixed mojitos. It will, that is, until the epidural starts to wear off, and suddenly you're at a much-dreaded work event, where the guest of honor is your nasty boss, and he's going to charge you for that drink.

Of course, none of the above is meant to say that childbirth *with drugs* is a walk in the park and childbirth *without drugs* is one stop short of hell, but if it becomes apparent that you really weren't paying attention in those expensive childbirth classes, then an epidural is one option at your disposal.

Another option is, of course, to actually pay attention in your childbirth classes.

Getting comfy in the hospital

How to take advantage of your temporary accommodations

Your hospital room—the one you will be just thrilled to collapse in shortly after the arduous process of bringing your baby into the world, despite the late-1980s dusky pink walls and yellow and mauve geometric-patterned easy chair—offers all kinds of free stuff of a personally enriching, emotionally satisfying nature. Cherish your time in this haven of relative luxury as trained professionals respond to your every whim, and be sure to use, borrow, steal, and enjoy whatever you can.

LIBERATE SMALL ITEMS OF A USEFUL NATURE. Like hotel rooms that offer miniature shampoos, body lotions, and shower caps, hospitals are full of stuff that you are expected to walk out with. These include but are not limited to receiving blankets, bulb aspirators, thermometers, baby wipes, little T-shirts (typically emblazoned with the hospital logo and the year, although not the current one), and tiny diapers. While most of the above is specifically intended for your child's health and well-being, there are some items just

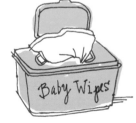

for you, such as exceptionally large 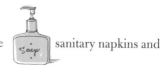 sanitary napkins and antibacterial soap by the gallon.

DEMO THE MOVEABLE BED. We've all seen and thoroughly enjoyed the infomercials on those cunning adjustable beds that can bend to raise you into a seated position so you may read or watch TV in comfort, or lift your lower legs for no discernable reason whatsoever. Great news—your hospital room will probably come furnished with something similar. So, once you've got though all that childbirth stuff, you can retire to a bed that can arrange your body into all kinds of interesting positions at the flick of a switch. This will prove to be quite handy, because you will probably be so exhausted that voluntary motion is virtually impossible.

SEEK HUMOR IN UNUSUAL PLACES. You will be able to derive enormous pleasure from watching your partner try to get comfortable on a tiny hospital cot while you effortlessly elevate your head and bend your knees in your aforementioned remote-controlled bed.

DRINK CHAMPAGNE IN BED. At least one or two of your visitors will rightly assume the thing you have missed most while being pregnant is a partaking of a beverage of an alcoholic nature. Without condoning excessive drinking while breastfeeding, it must be said that giving birth to a child is a wonderful opportunity to lie back, bask in the afterglow of your accomplishments, and knock back a small one while surrounded by a complimentary and awed crowd who hang on your every word. Disregarding the fact that you're wearing one of the hospital's heinous nursing nightgowns, it's the closest you'll ever get to that *I've-just-won-an-Academy-Award* feeling.

SURVEY THE SPOILS. Some people will come with gifts; others will bring flowers. Whatever the exact nature of the loot, enjoy being surrounded by goodies and the knowledge that they're all for you. Well, maybe the cashmere onesie and hat set is for your baby, but it's thanks to you that he'll have the pleasure of spitting up on it for weeks to come.

SEE WHAT IT'S LIKE TO HAVE A NANNY. It's reasonable to expect that, in the first couple of days after the birth of your baby, somebody else will be on diaper duty. Certainly, since you will be changing about a million of them over the next few years, it's important to delay the onset of this overrated activity for as long as possible. Also, remember (and remember to point out to others) that it's quite impossible to change a diaper while you're lying down. Make sure you stay in a recumbent pose for about forty-eight hours, or at least wait to stretch your legs until some nice nurse has been in and checked your baby, pronouncing him fresh and fragrant. This will in no way compromise your ability to connect with your baby on an emotional level. (Poop is not the glue that binds mother and child.)

FIND TIME TO RELAX. Your job, for the next day or two, is to rest up, wrestle with the knotty problem of breastfeeding an infant whose head is a fraction of the size of your boob, and watch daytime soaps. But somewhere in that busy schedule you may find time to catch up on a few of those little personal needs that got left by the wayside in the harried flurry of your final weeks of pregnancy. Remember, your hospital stay presents a great opportunity to give yourself a facial (those curiously shaped vomit receptacles are just the right size for combining oatmeal and mashed avocado); use the handily situated bedside telephone to call your friends (and tell them about your facial); and enjoy eating all your meals in bed without someone complaining about your getting crumbs (or, indeed, whole muffins) in the sheets.

GET ALL THE FREE ADVICE YOU NEED. Actually, nothing connected to the medical side of the whole pregnancy and birthing experience is exactly free—if you're not paying those exorbitant monthly health insurance premiums, you're submitting yourself to a boring job because it has a decent benefits package. In either case, you might as well make the most of your hospital experience. These places are just bursting at the seams with people desperate to give advice on the health and well-being of your child. So ask all the questions you want, taking copious notes if you have the presence of mind, and so avoid having to make multiple, costly appointments with your new pediatrician the week you return home with your new baby and find yourself entertaining raging fears concerning excessive snot and impossibly frequent pooping.

PRACTICE FOR PARENTHOOD. Just as you and your offspring are getting all snuggly together in your new room, you will be interrupted by nursing staff coming to look at your baby. They'll check his vital signs, examine his diaper, and review his milk intake, and they will perform this routine every couple of hours. While it's obvious that there are good reasons for this, the concept of night (i.e., sleeping) and day (i.e., being awake) is totally meaningless in a hospital environment. This will be highly annoying at first, but comfort yourself with the fact that, as soon as your baby perks up from his birthing exhaustion, he will be the one to stir things up. The nurses are, in fact, doing you a favor by easing you rather gently into a lifetime of disturbed sleep. At least, they tiptoe around your room, as opposed to wailing inconsolably, farting loudly, and demanding that you Take Your Top Off Right This Very Minute.

Meeting your friend's beautiful baby

What to say when it's most certainly not

Given the fact that you have just delivered the world's most beautiful baby, it stands to reason that any other infant you meet is going to be considerably less attractive. But meet them you will. As a new mom, you will likely spend the next few months greeting newborns—babies you encounter in the hospital or at your pediatrician's office, the offspring of your similarly fertile friends and coworkers, the children of the women in your mothers' group. And, quite naturally, you will be expected to make little cooing noises of delight over their children, just as they do over yours.

If polite enthusiasm isn't your strong suit—and after such a wonderfully self-centered pregnancy, you're probably a little out of practice—it's best to be prepared for these situations, and more important, for the possibility of being suddenly thrown off course by an unexpectedly ugly baby (not yours, of course).

First, have at your disposal a number of useful blanket statements like:

"He's so gorgeous."

"Isn't she beautiful?"

"What an amazing child!"

Any of the above can serve as an excellent starting point. Then, if you think you can pull it off, qualify your opening gambit with a statement that's more personalized and yet not untruthful, such as one of the following:

"Look at those cheeks."

"Her eyes are so blue."

"What a lot of hair!"

It's a good idea to have quite a few of these up your sleeve, so you can use the one that's most physically appropriate. There's no point in rambling on about golden curls if the child in question sports a single tuft of mousy fuzz. Take a moment to *actually look at the child,* and make sure that your repertoire includes options for all manner of babies—the good, the bald, and the ugly.

After establishing that you're both observant and thoughtful, you can move on with some general questions. Questions are good—they show that you are interested in your friend's baby but they do away with the unpleasant urge to tell even more barefaced lies. Good examples are noncontentious ones like these:

"How is he sleeping?"

"How's the feeding going?"

Better yet, compliment your friend's baby on temperament and personality attributes that suggest a unique level of intelligence, unusual in one so young:

"She seems so alert."

"Look how mellow he is!"

"Look how she's taking everything in!"

These kinds of statement work best if the child is awake. If the child is sleeping, try:

"I've never seen such a calm and settled newborn."

This is typically interpreted as a glowing testament to your friend's superlative mothering skills, and it will earn you many useful points in anticipation of the day you suddenly find you need a babysitter so you can use that soon-to-expire spa gift certificate you got at your shower.

Receiving undesirable gifts

How to be gracious as you unwrap your fourth diaper bag

It's sad to say, but you're probably going to spend the next twenty or so years of your life apologizing (with various degrees of success) for the things you child has or hasn't done. You should, therefore, start practicing your poker face now. Fortunately, the aftermath of childbirth gives you plenty of opportunities to feign sincerity.

Because you've just had a baby, legions of your babyless friends will stop by bearing gifts. As everybody knows, a new baby means presents, ostensibly for the baby but really for you, being that your baby couldn't give a hoot about anything that does not come in a nursing bra. And by a strange law known only to very new, very hormonal mothers, a full 76 percent of nonregistry baby gifts are either tasteless or useless. At this point, you're equal parts venom and breast milk, and it doesn't take much (the lack of a gift receipt, for example) to push you over the edge.

An unwelcome gift tends to fall into one of three main categories. Either it'll be ugly—this usually applies to clothing, although nothing is a lifetime commitment to a person who gains a pound every couple of weeks. Or it'll be a duplicate of an item you already have. Or it'll be something that comes with some kind of moral baggage, something that quietly signals a lack of faith in your abilities to look after a baby without scrutiny or advice. This last type of gift includes items such as:

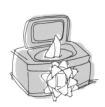

BOTTLES AND OTHER FEEDING EQUIPMENT. This gift says, "I think it's commendable that you're going to try breastfeeding, but we both know that you don't have the stamina or the patience, so you might as well go straight to formula."

BREAST PUMP, NURSING PADS, AND SO ON. This gift says, "Breastfeeding is the only way. That's what boobs are for. So don't let me catch you mixing formula."

WIPE WARMER. This gift says, "I can't believe that you'd be so cruel as to wipe your baby's bottom with a cold wipe straight from the tub. If you weren't such a good friend I'd be tempted to call the authorities."

PINK AND BLUE GENDER-SPECIFIC CLOTHING. This gift says, "I don't hold with this notion of dressing kids in nontraditional colors. It leads to wanton homosexuality, and when your child becomes a cross-dressing dominatrix, you will have only yourself to blame."

To deal with an unwelcome gift of any nature, simply follow this three-step program:

STEP 1:

PERFECT YOUR IMPRESSION OF A CALM
MADONNA-LIKE FIGURE.

Here you are, tired but happy, a morsel of a child at your breast,
sunlight streaming into the room, surrounded by flowers and
the other spoils of childbirth. You exude an air of tranquility
and entirely deserved self-satisfaction. Further the illusion by
opening every gift as if it were the next best thing to being handed
your perfect newborn.

STEP 2:

DEVELOP AN AMUSING CODE WITH YOUR PARTNER.

Even though you hate the gift, say something like "How
fabulous! I love it! Honey, did you remember to feed the cat?"
Incorporating a reference to a pet you do not even have is simply
your secret language for "How hideous! I hate it! Honey, did
you ever see anything quite so obnoxious in your life?" It's fun.
You'll see.

STEP 3:

ABOVE ALL, GIVE YOURSELF TIME.

Don't be harsh until you've had a chance to live with a gift and
discern its inherent usefulness or extremely well-hidden beauty.
Keep in mind, also, that most things can be re-gifted; that
duplicates can be useful because poop and puke gets everywhere;
that beauty is in the eye of the beholder (however blind to good
taste the beholder may be); and that you must never, ever alienate
a potential babysitter, and that means any adult of fairly sound
mind and reasonable reputation (and especially anybody who was
nice enough to give you a gift in the first place).

Postscript : Sharing your life with a baby

How to enjoy the perks together

The day that you thought would never arrive has come and gone. You have a baby. And that means you are no longer pregnant. After forty long weeks, it may seem quite an extraordinary state of affairs. You may even feel a little sad, especially if you had a fun pregnancy, and especially if your new baby is a live wire who needs about three minutes of sleep a day.

But it's time to move on. Your self-indulgent pregnant life is over, and your equally self-indulgent postpartum life is just beginning. For aside from the well-documented joys of parenthood, there are many benefits that come with your new situation. These include:

REFLECTED GLORY. Babies are truly amazing things, and the process by which they get into the world is also pretty miraculous. One day you have a big belly, and the next you have a big belly and a small baby. It's quite astonishing. Naturally, you deserve a lot of attention for performing this amazing feat. Although it may seem that your baby is the recipient of all the praise during the first few days and weeks after the birth, we all know that when people say, "Look at those cheeks!" what they really mean is "How on earth did you deliver such an enormous child? You go, girl!"

Remember, your new baby's accomplishments are actually your own. Gaining weight, acting cute, being able to wear red without looking sallow—it's all stuff in which you may take personal pride.

PERSONAL GIFTS AND FAVORS. While people love to shop for babies, there are always some who care not for teeny-weeny shirts and microscopic socks. These are the friends who come to visit your baby but bring you a gift like bubble bath or chocolate, and offer to babysit while you enjoy a nice long soak in the tub, a box of soft centers at your elbow.

FAVORABLE ATTENTION. Life with the exterior baby is really not so very different from life with the interior version. People still feel inclined to smile at you on the street, make room for you on public transport (sometimes), hold doors open for you, and generally treat you like the superior being you are. Enjoy this now, while your baby is small and compliant and has no opinion of his or her own. The general public is less kindly disposed toward the mothers of noisy and unappealing two-year-olds.

LICENSE TO GORGE. If you feel you need justification for continuing to eat like it's going out of fashion, there is no better reason than breastfeeding. When you're nursing an infant you need an extra five hundred calories every day—more than you needed when you were pregnant. And if you enjoyed eating then, just think about the damage you can do now. Breastfeeding is also, as you might have heard, a great way to lose weight over the long haul. And this statement, unlike "Most first labors are only about ten hours long," and "You'll probably have a small baby," is generally true.

PERMISSION TO ENJOY NEW ACTIVITIES. With a baby in tow, you can do all the things for which you never previously had the time or felt youthful enough. You can stop to sit and breastfeed in all manner of cozy locations, like those big armchairs in bookstores and coffee shops (while partaking of a small snack yourself, of course). You'll also gain a whole new circle of like-minded friends (your mothers' group, your baby music class, your fellow coffee-shop loiterers). Feel free to pay the exorbitant admission fees to theme parks, and hurry along to all the other places nominally designated for small children that you've been secretly itching to visit, like pet shops, mega toy stores, and zoos.

AN EXPANDED MUSIC COLLECTION. Playing classical music to your infant is said to stimulate the brain, promoting future intelligence, but who's to say that the same isn't true of 1970s disco classics or hip-hop? Having a baby gives you license to enjoy all things that come under the heading of Infant Stimulation—music, art galleries, movies. And what baby doesn't love an outlet mall?

MORE OPPORTUNITIES TO SHOP. Even if you took in a great haul at your shower, the wonderful thing about babies is that they keep on growing. Which means that you can keep on shopping. So although you may feel disinclined to buy new clothes for yourself (seeing as you're not *quite* at your target weight yet), at least

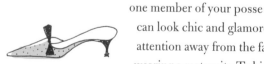

one member of your posse can look chic and glamorous (thus diverting attention away from the fact that you're still wearing a maternity T-shirt with permanent chocolate ice-cream stains).

UNCONDITIONAL LOVE; UNLIMITED SPIT-UP. Babies. They ooze mucus from all kinds of orifices. They projectile vomit or throw their food on the floor. They yell for no reason or, worse, answer back. They smile, and laugh, and giggle, and they're very generous with their hugs. They're temperamental, troublesome, fascinating, and amusing, and just spending every day of the rest of your life with Your Very Own Baby is undoubtedly the biggest perk of all.

ACKNOWLEDGMENTS

I wrote this book because I have such fond memories of being pregnant. I reveled in the attention, narcissistic being that I am, and was just fascinated by the forty pounds I gained around my middle. (I was somewhat less enthralled by it six months later, but there you go.)

Clearly, I couldn't have done any of it without the help of a couple of amazing babies, so thank you, Phoebe Rose Van Meter and Molly Frances Van Meter, exemplary and courteous tenants that you were. Their unintentional proficiency as babies-in-waiting most definitely gave me the inspiration to begin writing.

As I was in the thick of the bits about hospitals and drugs and epidurals, I was constantly reminded of the people who choose not to do it this way, for good reasons, and to their extreme satisfaction. My fabulous friends Kay and Joanna both had positive experiences of giving birth in nonhospital settings (like bathtubs), with midwives and without drugs. In this, as in most other things, I admire and respect them and can only wish that I wasn't such a big scaredy-cat myself.

I'd also like to acknowledge Lisa Campbell at Chronicle Books, a most delightful and intelligent young woman, who offered me the opportunity to write this book, and who edited it with a lightness of touch that I found both gratifying and flattering.

And finally, here's to Luke, the father of my children, who appears to have had something of a significant role in providing me with the source of my inspiration. Despite his persistence in referring to the writing of this book as *my hobby,* I have to say that he's a great dad and jolly nice chap. I love him immensely.

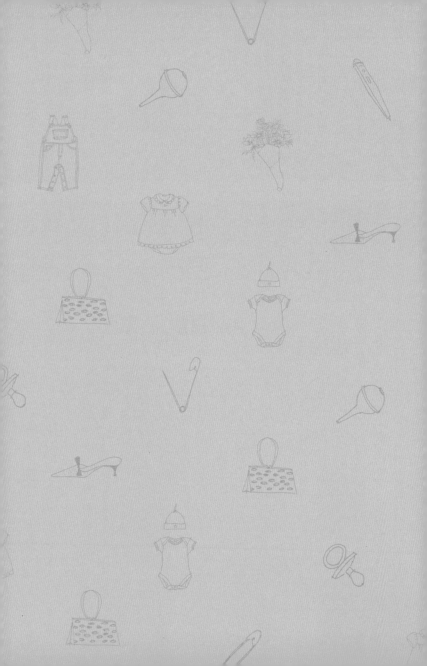